Second Edition

# CHILDHOOD VACCINATIONS

## ANSWERS TO YOUR QUESTIONS

Published by Inhabit Media Inc. (www.inhabitmedia.com)

Inhabit Media Inc.
(Iqaluit), P.O. Box 11125, Iqaluit, Nunavut, X0A 1H0
(Toronto), 146A Orchard View Blvd., Toronto, Ontario, M4R 1C3

References:
Bailetti, K. Childhood Vaccinations: Answers to Your Questions, Second Edition. Inhabit Media, Toronto, 2010.



Companion book to Childhood Vaccinations: Making Informed Decisions / Katia Bailetti. -- 2nd ed.

Printed and bound in Canada on recycled paper.

10 9 8 7 6 5 4 3 2 1

Library and Archives Canada Cataloguing in Publication

Bailetti, Katia, 1975-
Childhood vaccinations : answers to your questions / Katia Bailetti. -- 2nd ed.

ISBN 978-1-926569-13-0

1. Vaccination of children--Popular works. 2. Vaccination of children--Complications--Risk factors--Popular works. 3. Vaccines--Health aspects--Popular works. I. Title.

RJ240.B232 2010 614.4'7083 C2010-904843-1

Second Edition

# CHILDHOOD VACCINATIONS

## ANSWERS TO YOUR QUESTIONS

Katia Bailetti ND

INHABIT
MEDIA

## Disclaimer

This book is not intended to provide a complete overview of childhood vaccinations, nor is it a substitute for information and advice from your primary health care provider. Any decision regarding your health should be made in consultation with your health care provider. Readers are encouraged to continue to collect information about vaccines and discuss any questions or concerns with their doctor. The author, editors, and publisher assume no responsibility for any effects associated with making decisions about vaccinations or health care based on the information provided in this book. The opinions in this book do not represent the opinions of anyone other than the author at the time of writing. All efforts were made to ensure the accuracy of the information contained in this book as of the date of writing, but readers should be aware that medicine is a continually evolving science.

To *Kalah, Faron, Kiefer, & Danny*

# CONTENTS

# INTRODUCTION

My interest in childhood vaccinations began approximately ten years ago, after I heard about a severe adverse reaction to a vaccine in a previously healthy child. At that time, I had no idea that it was possible for vaccines to cause harm. The details of this child's story are described in chapter 2. Since then, I have been collecting information and research about childhood vaccinations.

I began to thoroughly research childhood vaccinations when I became pregnant with my daughter but the more I researched, the more overwhelmed and confused I felt. Every question I had led to more questions. Studies and health professionals often contradicted each other and much of the information available seemed to be written from a very polarized perspective. In addition, I was not sure whether the information I was gathering was applicable to the vaccines currently used. There were so many unknowns, but I was determined to study the subject of vaccination until I felt I was able to make sense of the various issues.

After our daughter was born, we received a vaccination schedule from our pediatrician and very little accompanying information. It was then I decided to organize the information I had collected to make it accessible for other parents struggling with their vaccination decisions. My own confusion and subsequent quest for answers became my motivation for writing this book and the accompanying workbook.

During my quest to find the answers to my questions about vaccines, I have felt conflicted: at times I have felt strongly for and strongly against vaccines. Although I now feel comfortable with our vaccination decisions, I cannot side with only one perspective and I am not the only professional who feels this way.

An increasing number of medical professionals, researchers, and parents are asking questions about childhood vaccinations. If you are one of these parents, you are not alone. A Canadian survey in 2001 found that 38% of parents with children under seven were not sure that vaccinations were beneficial. However, few parents who question the safety, efficacy, or necessity of vaccines are currently able to find answers. Many of these parents proceed with vaccinations because they are unaware of their options or because they feel an overwhelming pressure to conform. It is my firm belief that parents should be provided with the information they need in order to make informed decisions about their child's health care.

It is important to be informed about vaccinations and to clarify what is important to you, as a person and a parent. The aim of this book is to help parents feel more comfortable with their vaccination decisions and enable them to communicate concerns and views to doctors, family, and others.

## *Overview*

The topic of childhood vaccinations includes many different issues and perspectives. Through my many lengthy discussions with other parents, a number of common concerns have surfaced. The focus of this book is to address these concerns and help parents make informed decisions about their children's vaccinations with relevant, up-to-date, and reliable information (primarily from peer-reviewed medical journals and trusted government agencies).

The book is organized into three chapters: chapter 1 provides an introduction to vaccine basics, the infections they protect against and vaccination options; chapter 2 provides information about general vaccination issues such as safety and efficacy; and chapter 3 offers details about specific vaccination issues such as the vaccine–autism controversy. Each chapter begins with a list of key concepts and a complete list of references is included at the end of each chapter. Examples, data, and research presented are often North American, but the concepts are relevant for parents worldwide. As you read through this book, I encourage you to use the accompanying workbook to help you with the process of making your informed vaccination decisions.

## *Overview of Childhood Vaccinations: Making Informed Decisions (accompanying workbook)*

The workbook was created to accompany *Childhood Vaccinations: Answers to Your Questions*, however, it is not essential that these books are used together. The focus of the workbook is to help parents to make informed decisions about childhood vaccinations and to take readers through the step-by-step decision process. The workbook includes alternate vaccine schedules, recommendations to decrease your child's risk of a serious infection and vaccine complication, and information about how to gather accurate and relevant vaccine information. The workbook also offers worksheets, sample letters, and resources.

## *Vaccine Lectures, Consultations, and Support*

For additional information about upcoming vaccination lectures, consultations and resources, please visit my website at www.drbailetti.com

Chapter 1

# VACCINATION, INFECTIONS, AND OPTIONS

What is vaccination and how does it work?

What do we vaccinate against?

What is the recommended vaccination schedule?

What are my options?

How likely is an infection?

How likely is a serious complication?

Are treatments available for infections?

Who is at risk of becoming infected?

## Key Concepts

*Vaccines can offer some protection against infections.*

*Vaccinations usually begin within the first two months of age.*

*Vaccination options are available.*

*Some vaccine-preventable infections are typically mild, but all infections can result in serious complications.*

*Treatments are available for some vaccine-preventable infections.*

*Some children have a greater risk of being infected and developing serious complications than others.*

# VACCINATION, INFECTIONS AND OPTIONS

## *What is vaccination and how does it work?*

Vaccination is the administration of a vaccine into the body with the intent of protecting the body against a similar type of infection in the future. The active ingredient in a vaccine is usually a modified virus, bacteria, or toxin. Once these active ingredients are injected into the body, the immune system identifies them as foreign invaders, or antigens, and initiates an immune response. These active ingredients are weakened, or killed, by vaccine manufacturers to help stimulate an immune response without causing the actual illness. The immune system is an intricate system of checks and balances, which involves many different types of immune cells and various levels of protection. For an overview of our current understanding of how the immune system works, please consult an immunology text or refer to *Understanding the Immune System: How it Works* — a book by the U.S. Department of Health and Human Services available online for free from this website: www3.niaid.nih.gov/topics/immune-System/PDF/theImmuneSystem.pdf.

Ideally, vaccines stimulate a specific and long-lasting immunity so that if the vaccinated person later encounters a similar antigen, the immune system can easily identify and overcome it. A specific immune response includes the creation of specific proteins called antibodies, which become attached to specific antigens. For example, polio antibodies will become specifically attached to the polio virus. Long-lasting immunity involves the creation of memory cells, which help the body "remember" intruders and stimulate a more rapid immune response when the body encounters a similar virus or bacteria in the future. In most cases, once the body has overcome a naturally acquired infection, it will develop a specific and long-lasting immunity to that infection. It is therefore unlikely (but not impossible) that an individual will become ill from repeated exposure to the same virus or bacteria. Vaccines attempt to stimulate the immune system in a similar way to naturally acquired infections. The terms "vaccination" and "immunization" are often used interchangeably, but they are not synonymous. Immunization involves the body developing immunity to an infection while vaccination does not always result in a body's immunity.

Vaccination has been referred to as one of the most effective preventative measures in the history of medicine. The idea of intentional exposure to a weakened infection to protect against a more serious infection is brilliant.[1] However, this concept may not be new as there are reports of people in many different countries who have been practising some form of vaccination for at least a few centuries before the first vaccine, as defined by Western medicine.

## *What do we vaccinate against?*

The current pediatric vaccination schedules in both Canada and the US recommend vaccinating against the following infections:

**Diphtheria** is a throat infection due to toxins released by *Corynebacterium diphtheriae* bacteria. It can be transmitted from person to person by casual contact (being in close proximity to a sick person).

> *Key symptoms include a low fever and a very sore throat with greyish coloured patches of pus at the back of the throat, which cannot be easily removed. Some people develop mild or no symptoms.*

**Tetanus (lockjaw)** is a nervous system infection due to toxins released by *Clostridium tetani* bacteria, which is commonly found in soil, especially where livestock live. This bacteria has also been found in the dust from streets and hospital operating rooms. It can be transmitted from the soil to a person through a deep dirty puncture wound such as a rusty nail or a large sliver.

> *Key symptoms include stiffness and spasms of muscles. The jaw muscle is commonly affected, which is why tetanus is sometimes referred to as "lockjaw." Other muscles can also*

*be affected, which can cause changes in facial expression, posture, and movement. These symptoms usually appear days, or weeks after exposure.*

**Pertussis (whooping cough)** is a throat infection due to *Bordetella pertussis* bacteria. This infection is transmitted from person to person by casual contact and is very contagious. Previously, almost 100% of children were infected by pertussis by their tenth birthday. Pertussis, or whooping cough, is often difficult to differentiate from other similar conditions, therefore, it is likely underreported. This infection is typically less severe in adults and more severe in infants under six months.

*Key symptoms include severe repeated coughing that lasts for longer than two weeks. The coughing spells often end with a high-pitched "whoop" sound as the infected individual tries to catch their breath, but this sound is not necessarily heard in infants. Infants often vomit from coughing so hard. The symptoms begin approximately seven days after exposure and last three weeks to three months.*

**Poliomyelitis (polio)** is a viral infection caused by a polio virus and it affects the nervous system. Approximately a century ago, almost all children were exposed to polio. It is usually transmitted from animal to person or person to person through water contaminated with feces. Because of polio and other infections, it is important to wash hands well after changing diapers and to choose safe water sources to drink, especially when travelling. Over 90% of people have no symptoms at all.

*Key symptoms of a serious infection include muscle tenderness, spasm, weakness, or paralysis. Polio can also cause meningitis (key symptoms below). Meningitis from polio usually results in full recovery.*

**Haemophilus influenzae type b (Hib)** was the most common cause of bacterial meningitis in children before the vaccine was released to the market. It can also cause other serious infections such as pneumonia, epiglottitis (a severe throat infection), septicemia (a severe blood infection), and septic arthritis. Many healthy people carry Hib bacteria with no symptoms. In fact, prior to the Hib vaccine, most infants under five years were carriers of Hib bacteria. This type of bacteria is not highly contagious and usually requires close direct contact for transmission (kissing or chewing on a toy that has been just chewed on by another baby).

*Key symptoms of meningitis include headache, neck stiffness, pain when bending head down to chin, and a change in consciousness (drowsy, difficulty waking, or incoherent speech). Meningitis can progress rapidly so do not delay diagnosis.*

**Invasive Meningococcal Disease (IMD)** is a serious bacterial infection due to *Neisseria meningitides*, a common cause of bacterial meningitis in children. Various subtypes of this bacteria exist and vaccines are available for some subtypes (A, C, Y and W135), but not all. As with Hib, serious infections such as meningitis can occur. Many healthy people carry meningococcal bacteria and display no symptoms and it usually requires close direct contact for transmission.

*Key symptoms of meningitis are listed in the Hib section.*

**Invasive Pneumococcal Disease (IPD)** is a serious bacterial infection due to *Streptococcus pneumoniae* which is the leading cause of bacterial pneumonia, meningitis, bacteremia (bacterial infection of the blood), and acute otitis media infections (middle ear infections) in children. As with Hib and meningococcal bacteria, serious infections such as meningitis can occur. Many healthy people carry meningococcal bacteria and display no symptoms. Close direct contact is usually required for transmission.

*Key symptoms of meningitis are listed in the Hib section above. Key symptoms of bacterial pneumonia include a cough with mucous production, difficulty breathing, chest pain, high fever, and chills.*

**Measles** is a flu-like infection due to the measles virus. Measles is highly contagious and can be transmitted from one person to another through casual contact. Prior to the development of the measles vaccine, almost all children were infected with measles. Measles is contagious before the appearance of the rash.

*Key symptoms include a fever, red eyes, and a red itchy rash that begins on the head then spreads to the rest of the body. Tiny white spots can be found on the inside of the cheeks. A measles infection lasts four to seven days.*

**Mumps** is a viral flu-like illness accompanied by swelling of the glands. It can be transmitted from one person to the next through casual contact.

*A key symptom is swelling of the salivary glands on the jaw below the ears. People with mumps can pass the virus on to others before this symptom appears.*

**Rubella (German measles or three-day measles)** is a flu-like infection caused by the rubella virus. Rubella used to be a very common infection in children before the rubella vaccine was introduced. Rubella requires close contact between people for transmission and is often so mild that it may even go unnoticed. Rubella is contagious before the appearance of the rash.

*Key symptoms include a fever, red eyes, and a pink rash that begins on the head then spreads to the rest of the body. It lasts approximately three days.*

**Varicella (chicken pox)** is a flu-like infection caused by the varicella virus. As with measles, varicella is highly contagious, can be transmitted from one person to another through casual contact, and is contagious before the rash develops. This vaccine is relatively new and the infection is still common in childhood.

*Key symptoms include a fever and very itchy red rash with fluid-filled blisters that begins on the head or thorax and spreads to the rest of the body.*

**Hepatitis B (hep B or HBV)** is a viral infection of the liver which can be transmitted from one person to the next through direct contact with blood or bodily fluids.

*Key symptoms include jaundice (skin appears yellowish) and abdominal pain.*

**Influenza (seasonal flu)** is a nose and throat infection caused by an influenza virus. It can be transmitted from one person to the next through casual contact and is usually more frequent during the fall and winter months. The most common types of influenza viruses are A and B. Influenza viruses mutate and modify their appearance rapidly. This ability to change appearance and mutate so quickly stimulates the body to respond to a reinfection of the same virus, as if it were a new infection. The virus's ability to mutate rapidly is the reason the flu can be caught annually and also why vaccine manufacturers create new flu vaccines every year. The influenza virus is not to be confused with *Haemophilus influenzae* bacteria, which was incorrectly named. In April of 2009, outbreaks of a new influenza type A virus caught the world's attention: H1N1 or the "swine flu." The virus spread from human to human across the globe and was labelled by the World Health Organization as a pandemic flu. A pandemic influenza is a virus that is easily spread between humans and affects a wide geographical area. The severity of pandemics vary.[2] An influenza pandemic does not necessarily cause more deaths than seasonal influenza.

The overwhelming majority of cases of H1N1 reported worldwide were uncomplicated flu-like illnesses, however there was some concern that H1N1 could have mutated into a stronger strain and returned in a more virulent form. A H1N1 vaccine was developed and is recommended for high-risk groups (including children older than six months and under five years).

*Key symptoms of seasonal influenza are sore throat, cough, runny nose, fatigue, sore body and head, and often a fever. The most common symptoms of H1N1 are a cough and a fever. Infected people also typically experience the same symptoms of seasonal influenza. In severe cases of H1N1, deterioration occurs three to four days after the onset of symptoms and major complications can be rapid. Symptoms that indicate a severe infection include fast or difficult breathing, bluish skin, a rash, pain when pressure is applied to the abdomen or chest, dizziness, confusion, severe or persistent vomiting, dehydration, inability to wake from sleep and flu-like symptoms that improve but then return with a fever and worse cough.*

**Human papillomavirus (HPV)** is a viral infection that is passed from one person to the next through sexual contact. It is the most common sexually transmitted infection. There are over one hundred different types of strains of HPV. Some can cause genital warts, while others can cause cervical cancer if left untreated for years.

*Most women have no symptoms and are able to overcome the infection without treatment. Some women develop a chronic HPV infection and are unaware of this until they receive an abnormal gynecological test result. Other common symptoms may include genital warts. Very little is known about how HPV affects men.*

The US vaccination schedule currently recommends vaccinations against two additional types of infections:

**Rotavirus** is a viral infection of the digestive system. The rotavirus can be spread through contact with objects that have been contaminated with infected feces. For example, if your child is sick and you change your child's diaper but do not carefully wash your hands before handling a toy, the virus could be passed on to another child who handles the same toy.

> *Key symptoms include watery diarrhea that lasts three to seven days as well as a high fever and vomiting.*

**Hepatitis A (hep A or HAV)** is a viral infection of the liver. Hepatitis A can also be spread from one person to another through contact with objects, food, or water contaminated with feces because of inadequate hygiene.

> *A key symptom is jaundice (skin appears yellowish), however, many people have no symptoms at all.*

## *What is the recommended vaccination schedule?*

Children's vaccination schedules are continually being modified and differ from one state or province to the next. Individual doctors may at times make additional recommendations for their patients by suggesting they forgo some vaccines or obtain additional vaccines. In North America, vaccination begins within the first two months of age. Within one injection, there may be more than one vaccine. For example, the diphtheria, tetanus, pertussis, *Haemophilus Influenzae* type b, and polio vaccines are typically combined into a 5-in-1 injection and the measles, mumps, and rubella vaccines are combined into the 3-in-1 MMR vaccine. Consult your family doctor, pediatrician, or local public health department for up-to-date recommendations.

Table 1 summarizes the most recent national recommendations for children in Canada. Each province and territory has its own recommendations that are accessible through the Public Health Agency of Canada.[3] The US recommendations differ slightly and include two additional vaccines: the rotavirus vaccine (at two months) and the hepatitis A vaccine (at twelve months).[4] For the recommended vaccination schedule in the US and other countries, refer to the Resources section of this book.

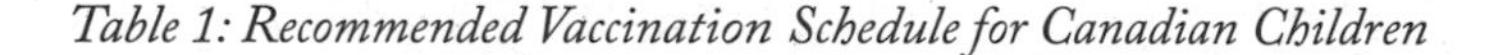
*Table 1: Recommended Vaccination Schedule for Canadian Children*

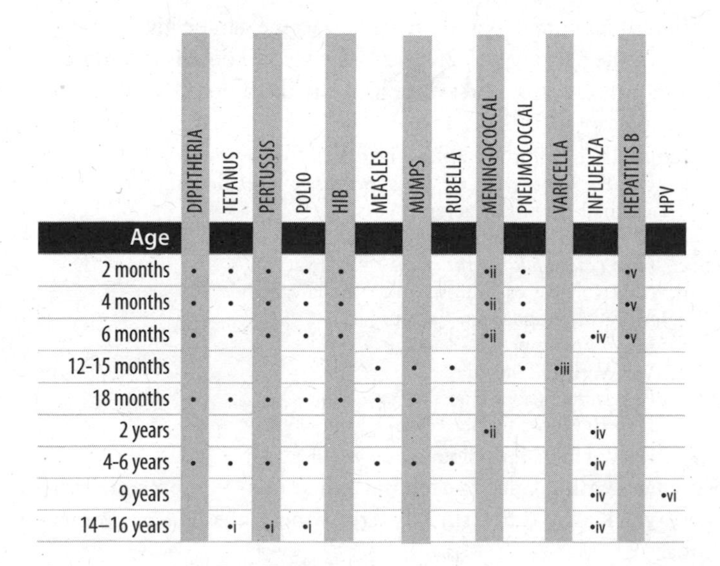

| Age | DIPHTHERIA | TETANUS | PERTUSSIS | POLIO | HIB | MEASLES | MUMPS | RUBELLA | MENINGOCOCCAL | PNEUMOCOCCAL | VARICELLA | INFLUENZA | HEPATITIS B | HPV |
|---|---|---|---|---|---|---|---|---|---|---|---|---|---|---|
| 2 months | • | • | • | • | • | | | | •ii | • | | | •v | |
| 4 months | • | • | • | • | • | | | | •ii | • | | | •v | |
| 6 months | • | • | • | • | • | | | | •ii | • | | •iv | •v | |
| 12-15 months | | | | | | • | • | • | | • | •iii | | | |
| 18 months | • | • | • | • | • | • | • | • | | | | | | |
| 2 years | | | | | | | | | •ii | | | •iv | | |
| 4-6 years | • | • | • | • | | • | • | • | | | | •iv | | |
| 9 years | | | | | | | | | | | | •iv | | •vi |
| 14–16 years | | •i | •i | •i | | | | | | | | •iv | | |

*Notes about the data:*

- Source: National Advisory Committee on Immunization and the Public Health Agency of Canada[5]
- i. At 14–16 years a booster is recommended that contains tetanus, diphtheria and pertussis or polio.
- ii. The meningococcal vaccine that is recommended is for one type of meningococcal bacteria labelled type 'C.' This vaccine can either be given at 2, 4, and 6 months or can be initiated at 12 months with a follow up dose during preteen years. Menactra, is a newly recommended vaccine against meningococcal types A, C, Y, W135 for high-risk groups. One dose of menactra is recommended for high-risk individuals and can be given anytime between 2 and 55 years of age.
- iii. Varicella vaccine can be given anytime between 12 months and 12 years.
- iv. The first influenza vaccine can be given once or twice within the first 6 to 23 months. Subsequently, it is recommended every fall. In addition, the H1N1 influenza vaccine is recommended for children 6 months to 5 years in one or more doses since they have been identified as a higher risk group. This information has not been added to Table 1.
- v. The hepatitis B vaccine can also be given during preteen or teen years in two or three doses.
- vi. The initial human papillomavirus vaccine can be given at any age between the age of 9 and 26 years. The second dose is recommended two months after the first dose and the third dose six months after the initial dose.[6]
- Vaccines are commonly abbreviated as follows:
    a. DTaP: Diptheria, tetanus, pertussis vaccine (the "a"'stands for acellular pertussis bacteria)
    b. IPV: Polio vaccine (inactivated/killed polio virus)
    c. Hib: *Haemophilus influenzae* type b vaccine
    d. MMR: Measles, mumps and rubella vaccine
    e. Men: Meningococcal vaccine
    f. Pneu: Pneumococcal vaccine
    g. Var: Varicella vaccine
    h. Flu: Influenza vaccine
    i. Hep B: Hepatitis B vaccine
    j. HPV: Human papillomavirus vaccine
- Provinces within Canada each have their own recommended schedules, which may differ slightly from the Canadian recommendations.

In some areas, proof of vaccination is required for daycare or school entry. Few parents are aware that exemptions are usually available for the required vaccines. For more information about exemptions, refer to the following section.

## *What are my options?*

Very few parents are aware they have vaccination options. Many presume or have been told that childhood vaccines are mandatory for children who attend school. In Canada, only three provinces require proof of vaccination against some infections for preschool and school entry. Ontario and New Brunswick require vaccines against diphtheria, tetanus, polio, measles, mumps, and rubella, for example, while Manitoba requires that children only receive the measles vaccine. In provinces where vaccines are required, exemptions are available for medical reasons, religious reasons, and reasons of conscience. In Canada, no childhood vaccine is mandatory. Requirements in the US vary from state to state. Contact your state's public health department for details. A summary of US exemptions can be found here: www.nvic.org/Vaccine-Laws/state-vaccine-requirements.aspx.

During a pandemic, mandatory vaccinations may be enforced in some areas or for some populations such as those at highest risk or those that provide an essential service such as health care.

What follows is an outline of three vaccination options to consider.

**Option 1:** Follow the recommended children's vaccination schedule. The benefit of this option is that parents can be assured that their choice is in accordance with what is recommended by various professional associations and committees. Parents will likely be fully supported by their medical doctor, and children who are vaccinated may develop immunity against some or all infections that they have been vaccinated against.

**Option 2:** Follow a modified vaccination schedule. This option requires that time is taken to work out a vaccination schedule with your doctor. Alternate vaccination schedules are outlined in the accompanying workbook *Childhood Vaccinations: Making Informed Decisions*. Some concerns about modifying the recommended schedule include:

- getting the vaccine before your child reaches the age when they are at the highest risk of being exposed to the infection;
- timing doses so they have a high probability of resulting in immunity;
- avoiding interactions between vaccines; and
- tracking the cumulative dose of other ingredients found in vaccines (e.g., aluminum).

Speak to your doctor about modifying the timing (delaying some or all vaccines or spacing out injections), reducing the number of vaccines given at one time, and selecting only some vaccines and avoiding others.

*Delaying:* The benefit of delaying vaccines is that it allows your child's body more time to develop on its own before adding vaccines which may affect the development of the immune system and nervous system. Children who are vaccinated later may also require fewer injections. The drawback of delaying is that some infections may be more dangerous in younger infants and delaying vaccines may increase your child's risk of one of these infections.

Women who are breastfeeding pass many immune-boosting components to their babies. If the mother has had one of these infections as a child, such as chicken pox, she will likely pass on protective antibodies for this infection to her child, which means her child has a lower risk of being infected with chicken pox while being breastfed. If a woman was recently vaccinated against chicken pox before pregnancy, she may also be able to pass on protective antibodies while breastfeeding.

*Staggering injections:* The benefit of increasing the time between injections is that it allows your child's body more time to recover. Recovery is especially important in children who have had reactions to vaccines in the past, children who are at a higher risk of suffering from reactions, or children who have symptoms of stress after they have been vaccinated. Stress symptoms include irritability, emotional instability, inability to concentrate, anxiety, being easily startled by sounds, grinding of teeth, stuttering, insomnia, diarrhea, changes in appetite, and nightmares. Staggering or spacing out injections must be discussed with your medical doctor because doses may have to be given within a certain period of time to maximize efficacy.

*Single vaccines and/or one injection per visit:* Combination vaccines are largely replacing single vaccines; however, a number of single vaccines are still available. It will likely be easier for a child's body to cope with a single type of vaccine (e.g., tetanus) at a time will than two multi-antigen vaccines. Single vaccines are ideal for those who have decided they only want a few vaccines. Single vaccines are also helpful for parents of sensitive children who choose to discontinue only the vaccine that has caused a reaction in their child. For example, if the diphtheria vaccine causes a problem, the tetanus vaccine boosters can still be given but separating combined vaccines into single vaccines will increase the cumulative amount of other vaccine constituents that are injected, such as aluminum. There may also be additional fees for single vaccines. Less vaccine safety information will likely be available for vaccines that are not commonly used. Opting to limit the number of injections given at one time will also inevitably increase the total number visits to the doctor.

*Selecting some vaccines and avoiding others:* Some parents decide to select the vaccines that offer protection against infections that their child is at high risk of coming into contact with, infections that are more serious, or those that are still affecting children in their country. Parents may also decide to omit the vaccines that protect against mild infections; vaccines that protect against low-risk infections and vaccines not required for school entry. The benefit of selectively vaccinating is that parents avoid some of the risks involved with vaccination. This option is popular with parents who have mixed feelings about vaccines, however, parents may have difficulties finding a health-care provider who will support this decision. Family, friends, and neighbours may even place pressure on parents to vaccinate for the safety of their own children (see the discussion on herd immunity in chapter 2). Whatever decision is made, be clear about reasoning and base decisions on current and relevant information. In order to feel more comfortable with your decision, you may decide to spend more time becoming familiar with signs and symptoms of serious infections. Regardless of your child's vaccination status, prompt medical assessment is recommended when your child has any symptoms that are of concern. Also, be aware of the legal process, as you may be required to obtain a formal exemption for your child to attend daycare or school. Exemption forms are available for medical reasons, religious reasons, or reasons of conscience. A medical exemption may be obtained from your medical doctor if your child has a contraindication to a vaccine, or a blood test shows he or she is already immune to an infection. A religious exemption may be granted if you belong to a spiritual organization which is against abortion as some vaccines are made from aborted fetal tissue. An exemption may also be obtained if your spiritual orientation does not allow the injection of animal or human products into the human body. In some US states, proof of affiliation with one of these religious organizations is required. Exemptions based on reasons of conscience or philosophical reasons are becoming more accessible to parents if vaccination is in conflict with a parent's firmly held belief. Refer to the Resources section for links to obtain exemption forms.

**Option 3:** Avoid vaccines altogether. The benefit of this option is the avoidance of nearly all of the risks associated with vaccination. Risk avoidance is significant since there is a lack of thorough understanding of vaccination risks, especially long-term ones and those associated with newer vaccines. All risks associated with vaccines are not eliminated because the health of unvaccinated people could be affected by the vaccinated people around them (for details, refer to the discussions on herd immunity and on the immune system in chapter 2).

Parents will likely have difficulties finding a health care provider who will support the decision to avoid all vaccines. Parents may also be opposed by family members, other parents, and school administrators. If parents proceed with this option, it is helpful to have a clear understanding of the reasoning behind it so that all communication with others about the decision is clear and straightforward. Please review the discussion of the previous option.

If you require assistance in exploring your vaccination options or would like support in making an informed decision, vaccine consults with health care professionals are available in Canada and the US (see the Resources section for details).

## *How likely is an infection?*

The risk of contracting most vaccine-preventable infections is low for the typical Canadian child, according to current statistics. The risk of contracting infections is likely even lower for people who are generally healthy, travel infrequently, live in smaller communities, and do not use large public transit systems.

It is difficult to estimate the true likelihood of contracting a vaccine-preventable infection because some of the infections are very mild, so medical help is not sought and the infection goes unidentified. Infections can also be misdiagnosed or not reported to public health officials. These statistics are only accurate when all health care providers report these infections to the Public Health Agency of Canada, as is required by law. Since these are the reported incidence rates, they do not represent the actual number of cases, however these statistics do provide a rough estimate. The most recent data available is included in Figure 1.

It is important to note that the incidence rate detailed in the data from Figure 1 does not distinguish between children who were previously healthy, versus those with underlying health conditions, nor does it distinguish between children who were previously vaccinated, versus those who were not. More specific information on these children's health conditions and their vaccination history would be helpful for parents who wanted to estimate their child's risk of contracting a vaccine-preventable infection.

Figure 1 reveals that the reported incidence rates of vaccine-preventable infections are low in Canada: less than one case per one hundred children in each age group. Since infection rates can increase and decrease over time, it is helpful to look at the average infection rate over a number of years as well. The average number of reported cases in Canada per year is available for some infections (calculated over five years from 2000 to 2004). The average for diphtheria, tetanus, polio, measles, mumps, and rubella is approximately zero cases per year. An average of one case of *Haemophilus influenzae* type b and ten cases of pertussis are reported per year in Canada.

Human papillomavirus infections are not currently reportable in Canada, therefore the number of cases in Canadian children is not available. The risk is very low for young children since HPV infections are typically transmitted by sexual contact. However, HPV infections can be passed

*Figure 1: Reported Incidence of Vaccine-Preventable Infections in Canadian Children in 2004*

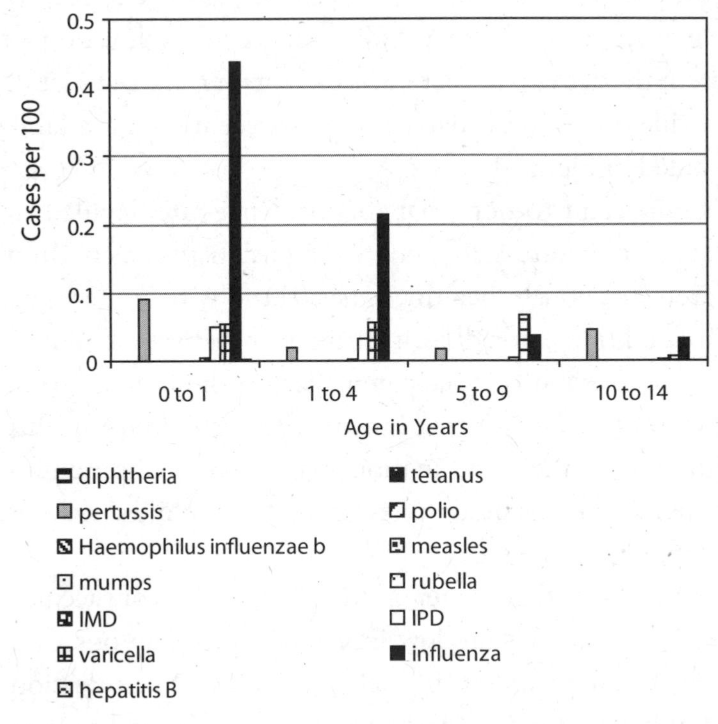


*Notes about the data:*

- Source: Public Health Agency of Canada[7,8]
- HPV is not a reportable infection in Canada, therefore its incidence is not included in Figure 1.
- The US schedule includes vaccines against two additional types of infections, which are not included in Figure 1.
- Figure 1 represents the reported incidence rates. The actual incidence of infection is likely higher for all infections.
- Viruses and bacteria have natural life cycles, therefore their incidence rates naturally increase and decrease over time. The data in Figure 1 is a snapshot in time; previous and subsequent years may have higher or lower incidence rates for each infection.
- Vaccination status and previous state of health is not considered in this data.
- For other data qualifiers, refer to the Public Health Agency of Canada.[9]

from mother to child through childbirth. Various Canadian population studies revealed that 3.4% to 42.0% of women were positive for a strain of HPV.[10] The highest incidence of infection is seen in adolescents and young adults (under 25 years).[11]

Assumptions may be made that the low rates of infection are due to a high vaccination rates in Canada; however, in 2004, few infants aged zero to two years old were vaccinated against influenza (4%) and pneumococcal bacteria (7%).[12] Low vaccination rates were also seen in the same age group for hepatitis B (14%), meningococcal (28%), and varicella vaccines (32%).[13] Some of these vaccines are relatively new, therefore, low infection rates cannot be attributed to a highly vaccinated adult population. This data may lead some to question the necessity of vaccinating every child in North America against all of these infections. It must be noted, however, that serious complications can result from virtually any infection (including the flu).

The new meningococcal vaccine recommended in Canada offers some protection against a variety of meningococcal strains (A, C, Y and W135). The average annual reported incidence between 1995 and 2006 of each type of invasive meningococcal infection found in the vaccine are as follows:

- A: 0.002/100,000 (median age was 48 and 2 cases were reported in 2006).
- C: 0.25/100,000 (median age was 19 and 43 cases were reported in 2006).
- Y: 0.09/100,000 (median age was 44 and 27 cases were reported in 2006).
- W135: 0.03/100,000 (median age was 19 and 6 cases were reported in 2006).[14]

By comparison, type B was responsible for 110 deaths in 2006 and the average annual incidence is 0.3/100,000 with a median age of 13 years.[15] Type B is not currently covered by the vaccine.

From the start of the H1N1 pandemic in the spring of 2009 to September 26th 2009, 1,479 people were hospitalized with H1N1 in Canada and 20% of cases were admitted to an intensive care unit.[16] The estimated number of people who died from H1N1 if they caught H1N1 (in the US) was very low (0.05%).[17] As of January 7th 2010 four hundred and fourteen people died due to H1N1 in Canada.[18] This falls well within the range of annual deaths due to seasonal influenza reported by Statistics Canada from 2003 to 2005 (data for later years are not yet available).[19, 20, 21] The Public Health Agency of Canada reports that the seasonal influenza virus typically causes 2,000-8,000 deaths per year in Canada (all ages).[22] The highest hospitalization rates were seen in children under fifteen years (10.4 cases per 100,000). The highest mortality rate was seen in people aged forty-five years and older (0.33 per 100,000). An underlying medical condition was present in 79% of the people who died.[23] As of September 6th 2009, the World Health Organization reported 3,205 deaths worldwide due to Pandemic (H1N1) 2009.[24] In comparison, the WHO estimates that 250 000 to 500,000 people die every year worldwide due to influenza viruses.[25]

## *How likely is a serious complication?*

Vaccine-preventable infections, which are usually mild or disappear on their own, include polio,[26] measles,[27] mumps,[28] rubella,[29] varicella,[30] influenza,[31] rotavirus infections,[32] hepatitis A,[33] and human papillomavirus infections.[34] Although there is limited information on the risk of a serious complication resulting from each vaccine-preventable infection, all vaccine-preventable infections can cause serious complications. This is especially true for very young infants, people who already have an underlying health condition and those whose immune systems are compromised. Below is a list of complications that may arise from vaccine-preventable infections. The frequency of each complication is included in the instances when this information is available.

**Diphtheria:** inflammation of the heart, kidneys, or the nerves.[35]

**Tetanus:** airway obstruction, respiratory arrest, heart failure, pneumonia, fractures, and brain damage.[36]

**Pertussis:** pneumonia, convulsions, seizures, nose bleeds, ear infections, brain damage (which can lead to learning and behavioural problems), bleeding in the brain, slowed or arrested breathing, and death. Approximately 20-30% of cases are admitted to a hospital, and 1 out of 400 cases admitted to a hospital ends in death.[37]

**Polio:** paralysis, disability or deformity, water in the lungs, shock, pneumonia, high blood pressure, urinary tract infections, kidney stones, loss of intestinal functioning, heart inflammation, and heart failure.[38] Note that over 90% of polio cases are very mild or go unnoticed and less than 1% of polio cases result in paralysis.[39]

**Haemophilus influenzae type b:** Hib bacteria can cause different complications based on where the infection is located. For those who develop Hib meningitis, death is a complication for 5% of cases and 15–20% have neurological complications such as hearing loss, seizures, brain damage, water on the brain, learning disorders, abnormalities in speech and language development, and behavioural problems.[40] Hib bacteria can also infect other parts of the body, such as lungs, blood, bones, brain, joints, and cause other complications.[41]

**Measles:** middle ear infection or pneumonia (10% of cases),[42] bronchitis, encephalitis (inflammation of the brain, 1 in 1,000 cases[43]).[44] Of those who end up with encephalitis, 15% die and 25% have persistent neurological problems.[45]

**Mumps:** infection of other organs including testes (20%–30% of post-pubertal males) and ovaries (in 5% of post-pubertal females), which rarely result in infertility, deafness (0.5–5.0 per 100,000 cases) and encephalitis (less than 1 per 50,000 cases).[46]

**Rubella:** encephalitis (1 out of 6,000 cases[47]), ear infection, transient arthritis.[48] Infections in the first ten weeks of pregnancy have an 85% risk of leading to congenital rubella syndrome, which can result in miscarriage and birth defects.[49]

**Invasive meningococcal disease:** In those who develop meningitis, complications include brain damage, shock, increased spinal fluid pressure, inflammation of the heart, water on the brain, deafness and paralysis.[50] Meningococcal bacteria can also infect the blood and cause other complications.[51]

**Invasive pneumococcal disease:** In those who develop meningitis, complications include water on the brain, deafness, paralysis, and brain damage.[52] Pneumococcal bacteria can also infect the lungs and cause pneumonia.

**Varicella:** secondary infection of the "pox" blisters (5%-10% of cases), encephalitis (1 out of 5,000 cases), low platelets (1–2%), hospitalization (2–3 per 1000 cases), uncoordinated walking (1 in 4,000 cases),[53] Reye's syndrome, pneumonia, inflammation of the heart, and transient arthritis.[54] Up to 2% of women who contract varicella during pregnancy give birth to babies with birth defects.[55]

**Influenza:** a wide variety of complications are possible including pneumonia, encephalitis, bronchitis, sinus infections, ear infections[56] and death.

**Hepatitis B:** liver cirrhosis (scarring of the liver) and liver cancer.[57]

**Human papillomavirus:** genital warts, cancer of the cervix or vulva in women.[58]

**Rotavirus:** severe dehydration and death.[59]

**Hepatitis A:** severe hepatitis and death.[60]

Measles, rubella, varicella, hepatitis B, and a number of other infections that are not vaccinated against can cause complications if a woman is infected during pregnancy. Complications range from low birth weight to birth defects and even miscarriage.[61] The risks appear to depend on the developmental stage of the unborn child at the time of infection. In general, the earlier the infection occurs during pregnancy, the higher the risk of complications. Some infections pose a lower risk (e.g., varicella), while for other infections the risk is higher (e.g., measles).[62] The benefits and risks of vaccinations before and during pregnancy, as well as during breastfeeding, will not be discussed here. It is important to note, however, that both infections and vaccine components can pass through the placenta and breast milk and affect the health of your child.

Many vaccine-preventable infections could result in death. Table 2 provides additional information about the number of children who have died from some of these infections in Canada over a two-year span (2004 and 2005).

*Table 2: Deaths Due to Infections in Canada in 2004 and 2005*

| | Total Deaths | | Deaths per 100,000 | | Deaths in Children aged 0-14 Years | |
|---|---|---|---|---|---|---|
| | 2004 | 2005 | 2004 | 2005 | 2004 | 2005 |
| **Influenza** | 296 | 678 | 0.9 | 2.1 | 3 | 1 |
| **Meningitis** | 53 | 53 | 0.2 | 0.2 | 12 | 14 |
| **Pertussis** | 0 | 1 | 0 | 0 | 0 | 1 |
| **Viral hepatitis** | 409 | 398 | 1.3 | 1.2 | 0 | 1 |
| **Meningococcal infections** | 14 | 13 | 0 | 0 | 3 | 3 |
| **Pneumonia** | 5,433 | 5,167 | 17 | 16 | 18 | 21 |

*Notes about the data:*

- Source: Statistics Canada [63, 64]
- Meningitis statistics are not specific to meningitis caused by Haemophilus influenza type B, pneumococcal, and meningococcal bacteria. The statistics also include deaths due to meningitis where other types of bacterial, viral, parasitic, fungal, and other infectious agents are suspected to be the cause.
- Pneumonia statistics are not specific to pneumonia caused by *Haemophilus influenzae* type b and pneumococcal infections. The statistics also include deaths due to pneumonia where other types of bacteria, viruses, fungi, and parasites are suspected to be the cause.
- Viral hepatitis statistics are not specific to hepatitis B. The statistics include all other types of viral hepatitis (e.g., hepatitis A, C and D).
- No children died due to polio or measles over the two-year span.[65,66]
- No data was provided by Statistics Canada for the following infections:
  a. Mumps, rubella and varicella, which are typically mild infections.
  b. Diphtheria and tetanus, which have very few, if any, cases every year in Canada.
  c. Human papillomavirus infections, which are thought to be the cause of approximately 390 deaths (in adults) in Canada in 2006.[67]

There were approximately 5,579,835 children in Canada aged zero to fourteen years old in 2006,[68] which means that the risk of a child dying from one of the above infections in 2004 and 2005 was estimated to be very slight (see Figure 2).

The infections included in Figure 2 rarely caused deaths in Canadian children in 2004. The information presented in Figure 2 is important to consider when reviewing other statistics that indicate the percentage of people who die out of all those who have contracted the infection (Figure 3).

*Figure 2: Deaths Due to Vaccine-Preventable Infections in Canadian Children in 2004*

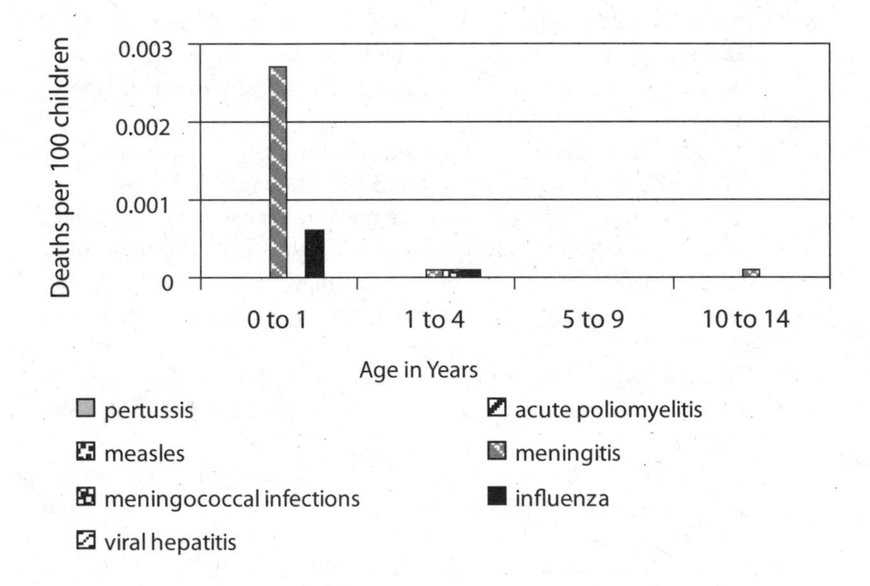


*Notes about the data:*

- Source: Statistics Canada[69]
- Death rates for diptheria, *Haemophilus influenzae* type b, mumps, rubella, pneumococcal infections, varicella, and tetanus were not included in Statistics Canada's mortality reports.
- HPV is not a reportable infection in Canada, therefore its death rate is not included in Figure 2.
- The US schedule includes vaccines against rotavirus, which are not included in Figure 2.
- Deaths due to meningitis include all types of bacterial meningitis, not only those due to *Haemophilus influenzae* type b, meningococcal and pneumococcal infections, for which vaccines are available.
- Deaths due to viral hepatitis include all types of hepatitis (i.e., A, C, D), not just hepatitis B.
- Vaccination status and previous state of health is not considered in this data.
- For other data qualifiers, refer to Statistics Canada.[70]

*Figure 3: Vaccine-Preventable Infections that Result in Death*

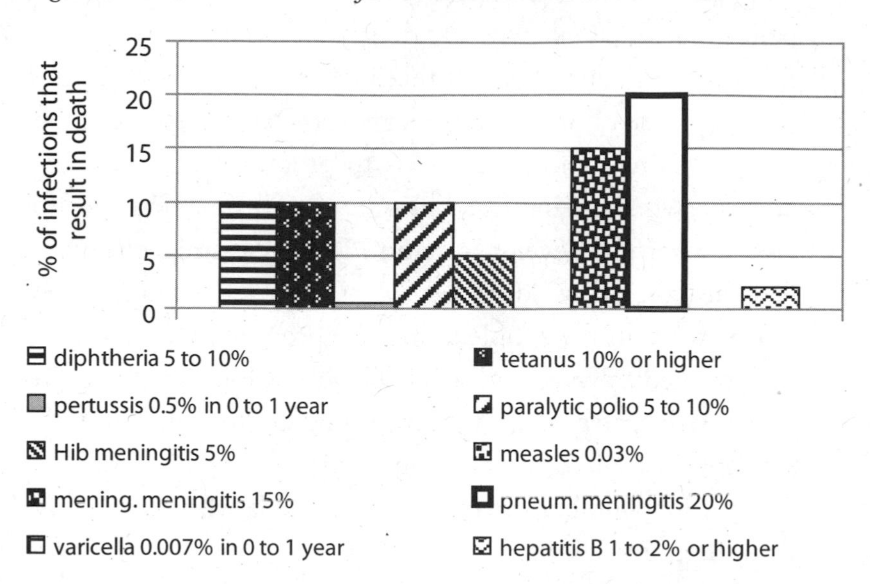


*Notes about the data:*

- Sources: Canada Immunization Guide (diphtheria, tetanus, polio, Hib meningitis, measles, varicella and hepatitis B),[71,72] Public Health Agency of Canada (pertussis),[73] National Library of Medicine and National Institutes of Health (meningococcal and pneumococcal meningitis).[74, 75]
- When a range of the percentage of infections that results in death is available, the graph reflects the highest percentage.
- Percentages were not found for the following infections: mumps, rubella, influenza, and HPV.
- Each percentage quoted may apply to a particular subgroup of the population (e.g., adults or infants under one year). Hib, meningococcal and pneumococcal vaccines protect against many types of invasive infections, including meningitis. However, percentages were only available for meningitis infections for each type of bacteria.
- Over 90% of polio cases are very mild or go unnoticed and less than 1% of polio cases result in paralysis.[76] Of the paralytic polio cases, the death rate is 5–10%.[77]
- Vaccination status and previous state of health is not considered in this data.
- The US schedule includes vaccines against two additional types of infections not included in Figure 3.

Figure 3 indicates that death is an outcome for a significant percentage of people who are diagnosed with diphtheria, tetanus, paralytic polio, and meningitis. What must be kept in mind is that it is uncertain how applicable these numbers are to children who have access to prompt health care and are otherwise healthy. In addition, the only data that specifically applies to a developed nation is the statistic for measles (1 death for every 3,000 cases).[78] Other data may or may not be relevant for people who have prompt access to high-quality medical care and are well nourished. To put these numbers in perspective it is important to keep in mind the very low risk of contracting one of these serious infections and the low number of children in Canada who actually die from these infections.

The statistical information presented here does not provide any background on the children's health status prior to infection. Children with a compromised immune system will have a difficult time recovering from any infection, therefore, they are at higher risk of serious complications.

To decrease your child's risk of becoming sick, refer to the recommendations outlined in Step 5 and 6 in the accompanying workbook *Childhood Vaccinations: Making Informed Decisions*.

## *Are treatments available for infections?*

Conventional medical treatments are available for some of the infections that we vaccinate against, but not all. Parents are often relieved to know that a medical treatment is available, but medications are not always effective. Likewise, parents can be especially concerned when there are no treatments available, but some infections that we vaccinate against are typically mild and require no medical intervention.

Antiviral drugs exist for varicella and influenza (seasonal and pandemic influenza H1N1). Antivirals do not exist for the other typically mild or self-limiting infections, which include polio, measles, mumps, rubella, rotavirus, hepatitis A, and human papillomavirus. Antivirals that do exist are not always available to everyone or at every hospital or clinic (especially in the event of a pandemic when there is a limited supply).

Medications are not usually needed for most HPV infections.[79] Some strains of HPV can cause cervical cancer, while others are more likely to cause genital warts.[80] Cervical cancer usually progresses very slowly and the vast majority of pre-cancerous cases can be easily detected and treated.[81] While surgery is available to remove large genital warts or early stage cancer cells, no antiviral medications are available.[82]

No medications are currently available for resolving hepatitis B infections either.[83] However, no treatment is required for most acute hepatitis B cases. Infections are asymptomatic in up to 50% of adults and 90% of children.[84] Infants who become infected with hepatitis B are, however, at a much higher risk of developing a chronic infection (90–95% for infants, 25–50% for children under five years) compared to adults (6–10%).[85]

A chronic hepatitis B infection increases the risk of developing liver disease and possibly liver cancer later in life.[86]

Antibiotics are available for the following infections: diphtheria,[87] tetanus,[88] pertussis,[89] *Haemophilus influenzae* type b,[90] meningococcal,[91] and pneumococcal.[92] Immediate treatment is usually recommended for these infections as treatments may not be as effective if they are not given promptly. Whenever a child has symptoms that are of concern, seek prompt medical attention regardless of the child's vaccination status.

In addition to conventional medical treatments, a variety of natural treatments are available. These natural treatments can help the body defend itself against bacterial and viral infections and improve the function of the immune system. The use of herbal medicine, homeopathic remedies, nutritional supplements, and other natural therapies can decrease the severity of infections, the risk of complications, and the total number of sick days. Consult a natural health care professional for details (see the Resources section).

## *Who is at risk of becoming infected?*

Children who are at a greater risk of getting sick from infections are those with an underlying health condition (either chronic or acute), those who travel to areas where there is a high incidence of infection, and those who are in close contact with an infected person such as a family member or friend. Children who are vaccinated may have a lower risk of becoming infected with the infections they are vaccinated against or of developing serious consequences (see the efficacy section in chapter 2 for discussion). Children who are breast fed for at least one year (exclusively for the first six months), offered a well balanced diet, exposed to fewer toxins, sleep well, relax often and are being cared for at home are at a lower risk of infection. Children who were not breastfed, undernourished, exposed to many toxins through their food, water, air and environment, often stressed and in a classroom with many other children are at a higher risk of infection as all of these factors significantly impact the ability of the immune system to function optimally.

Each of the vaccine-preventable infections can be transmitted from one person to the next through casual contact (sneezing, coughing, or shaking hands) except for tetanus, hepatitis B, and human papillomavirus.

HPV infections are sexually transmitted. Tetanus bacteria is commonly found in soil and tetanus infections are usually associated with deep, dirty puncture wounds. Hepatitis B infections usually occur in adults because contact with blood or bodily fluids is required in order to pass the infection from one person to another. However, it is important to remember that if infants are infected, they have a very high chance of becoming chronic carriers and are therefore at a higher risk of liver disease and liver cancer. There is conflicting information about whether the hepatitis B virus can be passed on from one person to the next through saliva. The confusion may be because some saliva can be contaminated with blood due to a slight cut or open sore somewhere in the mouth.

Below is a summary of conditions or situations that increase the risk of each infection as well as a list of high-risk groups. No specific risk factors were found for pertussis, measles, mumps, or rubella.

**Diptheria:** travel to high-risk areas[93] (see Resources section for travel information).

**Tetanus:** puncture wound, especially if there is soil in the wound.[94] Therefore, infants who are not walking outside unsupervised are at a low risk. However, 27% of cases in North America occur in people who do not report any injury.[95]

**Polio:** travel to high-risk area[96] (see Resources section for travel information).

**Haemophilus influenazae type b meningitis:** recent ear, throat or sinus infection; aboriginals;[97] children in full-time daycare (risk of infection is at least twice as high); and people with a spleen dysfunction or cochlear implant.[98]

**Invasive meningococcal disease:** close contact with infected family members or friend[99] including sharing utensils or kissing; people with a spleen that is absent or not functioning well; people with an immune system deficiency; travellers to places where the meningitis vaccine is required; research and laboratory personnel who are routinely exposed to *N. meningitides,* and military recruits.[100]

**Invasive pneumococcal disease:** children under two years; people over sixty-five years; people with weakened immune systems due to illness or medications (including people with HIV, sickle cell disease, diabetes); people with serious problems with the heart, lungs and kidneys; and anyone without a spleen or with a spleen that is functioning poorly.[101]

**Varicella*:** people who use medications over long periods of time (e.g., salicylic acid); have cystic fibrosis, are immunocompromised, health care workers and students; or susceptible household contacts of immunocompromised persons who cannot be immunized.[102]

**Influenza:** people over fifty; children between six months and two years; women more than three months pregnant during the flu season; anyone living in a long-term care facility; anyone with chronic heart, lung, or kidney conditions; anyone who has diabetes or weakened immune system apply to seasonal influenza.[103] People who were at highest risk of H1N1 influenza included people over sixty-five years; children under five years; people under eighteen years who are receiving long-term aspirin therapy; pregnant women; people with a chronic lung, heart, liver, blood, immune, neurologic, muscular, or metabolic disorders; residents of nursing homes and other chronic care facilities.[104] Research revealed that people who had previously been vaccinated for seasonal influenza may have been at higher risk of catching pandemic influenza H1N1.[105]

**Hepatitis B:** the child of a mother who is hepatitis B positive; a child-care setting where there is an infected child; exposure to contaminated blood or body fluids; unprotected sexual contact; injection drug users; hemodialysis patients; staff and inmates of correctional facilities; people who are immunocompromised; people who live in the same house as someone who is hepatitis B positive; who travel to a high-risk area; who have a chronic liver disease; people on hepatotoxic medications; and people who have undergone hematopoietic stem cell transplant.[106]

**Human papillomavirus:** people who have had sexual contact at an early age and people who have had multiple sexual partners; people who regularly use tobacco, drink alcohol or are chronically stressed; and people who have other viral infections, such as HIV and herpes.[107]

**Rotavirus:** the very young; the elderly; and those with a suppressed immune system.[108]

**Hepatitis A:** people living in a nursing home or rehabilitation centre; people who have a family member with a recent hepatitis A infection; intravenous drug use; and people who have recently travelled to Asia or South or Central America.[109]

*Provinces differ in their definitions of high-risk groups for varicella infections. Ontario risk factors are included here.

Chapter 2

# GENERAL VACCINATION ISSUES

Are there risks associated with vaccines?

What is in childhood vaccines?

Are vaccines safe?

Who should not be vaccinated?

Are vaccines effective?

What about herd immunity?

Does vaccination pose ethical questions?

## Key Concepts

*There are risks associated with vaccines.*

*Vaccines contain ingredients that can be hazardous to human health.*

*The current process for evaluating vaccine safety is not ideal.*

*There are some children who should not be vaccinated.*

*Vaccines can be effective, but do not guarantee immunity.*

*Your child's health and vaccination status can impact other people.*

*There are ethical concerns regarding vaccine delivery to the public.*

# GENERAL VACCINATION ISSUES

## *Are there risks associated with vaccines?*

Many people are unaware that there are risks associated with vaccines. I first became aware of the possible risks over ten years ago when a good friend of mine, Sonja, explained to me why she decided to discontinue vaccinating her children:

> *Kiefer was eighteen months old and it was time for his next diphtheria-tetanus-pertussis shot. The doctor told me that he may have a slight fever after the shot and to give him Tylenol. I remembered slight fevers and crankiness with previous shots in both my kids. No one told me about the possibility of other reactions.*
>
> *After his shot, Kiefer did have a fever. I gave him liquid Tylenol to help keep the fever down, but it did not help. He got hotter and hotter and was sweating and crying. He*

*finally fell asleep. In the middle of the night, he started crying and he was soaking with sweat and very hot. I couldn't wake him up; he just kept crying. Later, he was laughing and babbling. Then he had a seizure. I immediately called 911. The ambulance took us to the hospital where they gave him a rectal dose of acetaminophen. When he finally came out of his unresponsive state, he started screaming in a high-pitched tone, as if he was terrified or in severe pain. It was horrible and I couldn't calm him down. Eventually, he settled and a few hours later we went home. He was cranky for a few days. There was no explanation and no follow up. I never immunized either of my kids again.*[1]

Note: *This adverse reaction was prior to the removal of thimerosal from children's vaccines in Canada (in 1996)*[2] *and prior to the switch to the acellular pertussis vaccine DTaP (in 1997/8), which appears safer and more effective than the previous vaccine which contained whole cell pertussis.*[3]

Sonja's story initiated my interest in childhood vaccination issues. When I heard her story, I had just finished my training as a paramedic and Kiefer's mother had been working as a nurse for a few years. Neither of us knew that vaccinations could cause serious complications. Since then, I've heard many more accounts of serious complications following vaccinations from concerned parents who had no idea that there were risks involved. Many of these accounts were not reported and not all of the stories ended well. There are risks associated with vaccines. The complications can be serious and occur following a series of uneventful vaccination visits.

Despite these reactions, the majority of children in the US, Canada, and many other countries are being vaccinated and most appear not to suffer any serious complications immediately following vaccinations. However, there are a number of limitations within the current safety evaluation (refer to the safety section later in this chapter for details).

In an ideal situation parents would be able to estimate the probability that their child might suffer from a serious reaction as a result of each vaccine. Unfortunately, this information is not currently available. According to the Public Health Agency of Canada, the average rate of adverse reaction of any vaccine is 1 in 100,000 vaccines distributed.[4]

Some information about adverse reactions can be obtained from vaccine monographs posted online by vaccine manufacturers. Refer to the Resources section for links to vaccine manufacturers websites. Randall Neustaedter's book, *The Vaccine Guide: Risks and Benefits for Children and Adults,* is also a good resource, which identifies additional vaccine complications reported with each type of vaccine. The Vaccine Adverse Event Reporting System (VAERS) can be a valuable source of information as well. VAERS is a publicly accessible database, which collects reports of vaccine complications in the United States. Reporting is voluntary, so underreporting is one of the main limitations of the data. The data also includes coincidental events as well as complications truly caused by vaccines. My own search of the VAERS database revealed that in 2008, 315 reports of deaths and 595 reports of life-threatening events following vaccination in children aged zero to fourteen were filed. The vast majority (240 deaths and 315 life-threatening events) occurred in infants zero to six months of age. Canada also has an adverse vaccine reaction database, but it is not publicly accessible. A summary of more commonly seen adverse reactions was presented by the Public Health Agency of Canada in their 2006 Vaccine Safety Report. A total of 3,625 reports of complications from vaccinations were filed in Canada following vaccinations administered in 2004.[5] The types of complications ranged from minor reactions to life-threatening ones. Between 1992 and 2004, there were eight reports filed of deaths following vaccinations.[6] These reports were reviewed and three of the eight deaths were later attributed to a vaccination.[7] In each case, infants were involved but the vaccine in question was not part of the recommended children's vaccination schedule. Table 3 is a summary of some of the complications from vaccines that were reported in Canada in 2004.

*Table 3: Reported Reactions to Vaccines in Canada in 2004*

| | |
|---|---|
| **Minor Reactions** | • minor local reactions<br>• low fever<br>• conjunctivitis (pink eye)<br>• irritability<br>• headache<br>• nausea<br>• cough |
| **Moderate Reactions** | • severe pain and/or swelling at injection site<br>• allergic reactions (excluding anaphylaxis)<br>• high fever<br>• joint pain or arthritis<br>• oculo-respiratory syndrome (difficulty breathing, red eyes, and facial swelling)<br>• anorexia<br>• myalgia (muscle pain) |
| **Severe Reactions** | • anaphylaxis (serious allergic reaction)<br>• hypotonic-hyporesponsive episode (decreased tone of |

muscles and decreased responsiveness)
- localized anesthesia/paresthesia (loss of sensation or irregularity in sensations)
- thrombocytopenia (low blood clotting factor)
- Guillain Barré syndrome (an autoimmune disorder that causes paralysis)
- cranial or facial paralysis (e.g., Bell's palsy)
- meningitis or encephalitis (brain inflammation)
- screaming episode/persistent crying
- chest pain
- somnolence (abnormal sleepiness)
- hypokinesia (slow or few movements)
- dyspnea (difficulty breathing)
- convulsions or seizure
- death[8]

The risk of a severe reaction to vaccines appears to be low, however, it is impossible to have an accurate estimate of the risk at this time for the following reasons:

- No data on how many vaccines are administered to children in a given year is available. The rate of vaccine reactions is currently being calculated using the total number of vaccines distributed. The number of vaccines distributed is likely higher than the total number of vaccines administered since vaccines can expire before being used. Therefore the actual incidence rates of vaccine reactions are likely higher than the current estimates.
- More than one injection is often administered during a single vaccination visit, which makes it difficult to isolate which reactions are due to a single vaccine versus a reaction to a combination of vaccines. Administering more than one vaccine at a time is especially confusing when parents delay the start of their child's vaccination

schedule and then follow the recommended catch-up schedule. For example, if a child in Ontario has not yet received any vaccines by the time he or she reaches one year of age, the current recommendations is that the child receive five different injections, which is a total of eleven different types of vaccines in one day.[9]

- Reporting complications due to vaccinations is not mandatory everywhere, so it is likely that some reactions are not reported. In the few places where reporting is mandatory, it may not be enforced. Some reports of complications are incompletely filled out and therefore dismissed.

In addition to the reported complications, there is significant concern regarding the possible connection between vaccines and developmental disabilities (including autism), autoimmune diseases, inflammatory conditions, sudden infant death syndrome, infections, and other conditions (refer to chapter 3 for details).

Specific data on the incidence of vaccine complications must be made available before stating that the benefits of childhood vaccines greatly outweigh the risks.

To decrease your child's risk of a severe vaccine complication, speak to your naturopathic doctor about natural vaccine support and refer to the recommendations in Step 5 of the accompanying workbook *Childhood Vaccinations: Making Informed Decisions.*

## *What is in childhood vaccines?*

A list of vaccine ingredients can be found in vaccine package inserts and online monographs. Since some vaccine ingredients are considered proprietary information,[10] neither parents nor doctors have access to a complete list of all the vaccine ingredients. This lack of full disclosure is unfortunate, especially for people with a history of an allergic reaction to a chemical, those with a health condition that makes them more susceptible to damaging effects of chemicals, and people who are simply concerned about what is injected into their body. Childhood vaccines can contain heavy metals, such as mercury and aluminum; common allergens, such as soy, egg protein, monosodium glutamate, or MSG; antibiotics, such as neomycin; human and animal products, such as bovine serum, chick embryo, and human albumin; and other chemicals such as formaldehyde, 2-phenoxyethanol; as well as other undisclosed ingredients.[11]

The presence of allergens and antibiotics is relevant for people who have severe allergies. Antibiotics can also remove the body's protective "friendly bacteria" resulting in an increased susceptibility to infections and other health problems. Friendly bacteria can be replenished by using specific foods and probiotic supplements (speak to your health care professional for details). Formaldehyde is a cancer-causing agent[12] and aluminum and mercury can be hazardous to human health (refer to chapter 3 for details). Although only a very small amount of each of the previously mentioned components may be found in a vaccine, the long-term impact of injecting all of the components found in all childhood vaccines into infants has not been determined.

## *Are vaccines safe?*

The systems in place to maximize vaccine safety include regulatory bodies, clinical trial requirements for licensing, postlicensing surveillance, and research. For more information, please review vaccine safety information from the Public Health Agency of Canada at: www.phac-aspc.gc.ca/im/vs-sv/caefiss-eng.php or the Centers for Disease Control and Prevention www.cdc.gov/vaccinesafety/basic/safety.htm. In spite of these checks and balances, a number of safety issues remain. The following information is not meant to dismiss the efforts made by these organizations, but simply to point out that there are still a number of issues with vaccine safety. These issues include the following:

- Underreporting of vaccine complications. Only a fraction of the actual complications are reported by physicians to proper authorities. One study revealed that the underreporting of known complications to vaccines ranged from less than 1% to 72% in the US, which highlights the limitation of this type of surveillance in measuring the risk of adverse events.[13] If the conditions that have already been identified as vaccine complications are not being reported, it is unlikely that many of the conditions that have not yet been accepted as vaccine complications will be reported. The reporting guidelines clearly state that "any severe, unusual or unexpected event"[14] following vaccination should be reported. The lack of mandatory reporting requirements and a lack of serious consequences for physicians who do not report does little to alleviate the problem of underreporting. In Canada, only four provinces have mandatory reporting requirements for complications following vaccines.[15] Parents are generally unaware of their ability to report vaccine complications in the event that their doctor does not. The more reports of complications that are filed, the more information the medical community and the public will have regarding the risks associated with vaccinations. Refer to the Resources section for links to report a vaccine complication.

- Safety studies are not ideal due to the following reasons:

a. Prelicensing safety trials are usually limited in size. The regulatory body for vaccines in Canada requires just a few hundred subjects for each of the four phases of clinical vaccine assessment,[16] which leaves much of the safety assessment to be determined after licensing, since the less common adverse reactions will not be revealed by small studies.

b. Lack of long-term safety studies. Long-term safety studies are important in order to detect complications from vaccines that are not apparent shortly after vaccination. A vaccine may instigate a functional change in the body, but this change may not manifest itself as a significant sign or symptom for months or years. By the time the resulting medical condition is labelled by a medical professional, months or years may have gone by since the last vaccination. Therefore, each vaccine should be evaluated with a long-term safety study. In addition, there should be long-term studies that evaluate the safety of administering the combination of all the recommended childhood vaccines. The cumulative effect of administering all vaccines into the same child has not been evaluated.

c. Few randomized placebo-controlled trials. Research participants are randomly divided into two groups and one group receives an injection with a substance that is known to be safe, such as saline solution, while the other group receives the vaccine. This type of research provides the most reliable and valid evidence relating to vaccine safety, however, these trials are not done for all vaccines.[17] Instead of being injected with a saline solution, the control group is often injected with another type of vaccine. If there is no significant difference in the incidence of severe reactions in both groups, one could erroneously assume that the new vaccine is safe. The focus of this type of research is not to establish that a new vaccine is safe to use, but to establish that the new vaccine does not cause significantly more harm than another vaccine. In addition, randomized placebo-controlled trials that are carried out are not large enough to detect rare adverse events.[18]

d. Source of funding for safety research may influence results. Safety studies that are funded by organizations and associations with a vested interest in the results may not provide an accurate assessment of the real safety risks (refer to the Ethics section later in this chapter for discussion).

e. Lack of independent vaccine safety evaluation. Ideally, postlicensing safety surveillance should be designed and carried out by an independent organization whose members have no association with promoting vaccinations, vaccine manufacturing, or distributing compensation for vaccine injury. This would increase the likelihood that vaccines will be objectively assessed for safety. Safety studies that are funded by organizations and associations with a vested interest in the results may not provide an accurate assessment of the real safety risks. The Canadian Medical Association recently published a paper revealing the connection between industry funding and research results. The author concluded that "industry funding has a significant influence on the results of both surgical trials and drug trials."[19] A separate study published by the *British Medical Journal* revealed that "research sponsored by the drug industry was more likely to produce results favouring the product made by the company sponsoring the research than studies funded by other sources."[20] The source of research funding is not always included in published research papers, which makes it difficult to determine which studies are funded (directly or indirectly) by the vaccine industry.

f. Lack of relevant toxicity guidelines. There is a lack of specific guidelines for the safe injection in infants and children of all of the potentially toxic substances in vaccines. In some instances, the safety of a potentially toxic substance is assumed based on research that examines the safety of issuing vaccines only under the following conditions:

i) administering a similar substance, not the substance common to children's vaccines;
ii) administering the substance by mouth and not by injection;
iii) administering the substance to an adult or animal subject, not a human infant; or
iv) administering the substance on a short- term basis only.

Specific guidelines based on relevant research are needed for every component in vaccines that is known or suspected to be toxic to humans. Since the components in vaccines are injected together, guidelines for the safe injection of the combination of these potentially toxic components needs to be determined.

Specific guidelines are especially important for the following individuals:

i) premature infants;
ii) children who have conditions that make it difficult for them to eliminate toxins (e.g., kidney or liver conditions);
iii) children who receive additional vaccines (e.g., for travel); and
iv) children who have already been exposed to significant amounts of toxic substances, (e.g., children fed intravenously are already exposed to higher levels of aluminum).

## *Who should not be vaccinated?*

If your child has a health condition that is listed as a contraindication, he or she should not be vaccinated. If your child has a health condition listed as a caution, he or she may be at a higher risk of a severe complication from the vaccine. Contraindications and cautions associated with vaccines may be overlooked, especially during mass vaccination campaigns where medical charts are not available to the person administering the vaccine. Below is a list of general contraindications and cautions that apply to all Canadian vaccines. Each individual vaccine may have additional contraindications and cautions. These should be reviewed with your medical doctor before vaccinating.

*Table 4: Contraindications and Cautions to Canadian Vaccines*

| | |
|---|---|
| **Contra-indications** | • Anaphylactic reaction to a component of the vaccine<br>• Significant immunosuppression (for live vaccines only, e.g., the measles-mumps-rubella vaccine)<br>• Pregnancy (for live vaccines only) |
| **Cautions** | • Chronic underlying illness<br>• Compromised immune system<br>• History of Guillain-Barré syndrome with onset within 8 weeks of vaccination<br>• Recent administration of blood product containing antibodies (for a live vaccine only)<br>• Recent administration of live virus vaccine (for a live vaccine only)<br>• Severe bleeding disorder[21] |

The list of general contraindications includes a serious allergic reaction to a component of the vaccine.[22] However, since some ingredients are considered proprietary information,[23] there is no complete list of vaccine ingredients available to the public or to doctors. Therefore, parents cannot be absolutely certain of what is in each vaccine. Nevertheless, it is important to review the list of cautions and contraindications for each vaccine with your child's doctor prior to vaccinating as it will decrease your child's risk of suffering a serious complication. In addition to the cautions previously stated, there are a few additional cautions that are important to consider. These cautions include the following:

- Current infection or recovering from a recent infection,[24] since the body's immune system may already be working very hard.
- Premature birth, as the organs of premature babies may not be functioning optimally. Consider delaying first

injection until two months after the expected due date.

- Multiple chemical sensitivities or a family history of such sensitivities (due to the unknown ingredients in vaccines).
- Previous serious allergic reaction or family history of reactions (due to the unknown ingredients in vaccines).
- Immune system conditions or a family history of immune conditions (since vaccines may have a negative impact on the immune system, refer to the immune system section in chapter 3 for details).
- Neurological conditions or a family history of neurological conditions (since vaccines may have a negative impact on the nervous system, refer to the autism and mercury sections in chapter 3 for details).
- A health condition that affects the function of the kidneys, intestines, or liver (since all are required to remove potentially toxic vaccine components).
- A current health condition of unknown origin such as Kawasaki disease and systemic lupus erythematosus or recently recovering from a health condition (since the body's immune system may not be functioning optimally).
- Previous significant exposure to aluminum or mercury, including before birth (see the mercury section in chapter 3 for details).
- Pregnancy (for any vaccine containing mercury or aluminum or any other potentially toxic ingredient that may be passed to the unborn child through the placenta and breast milk).

## *Are vaccines effective?*

Public health agencies worldwide have reported that introducing a vaccine decreases the likelihood of infection, the severity of the infection, or both. There is some debate about how much of an impact vaccines have had on improving the health of highly vaccinated populations. For example, Dr. Sherri Tenpenny, who has practised emergency medicine in the US for over a decade and is the author of many vaccination books including *Vaccines: The Risks, The Benefits, The Choices,* has concluded that vaccines are not solely responsible for the elimination of infectious diseases.[25] Catherine Diodati is another vaccination authority who authored the book *Immunization: History, Ethics, Law and Health.* She concluded that vaccines have had little overall effect "upon mortality because disease related mortality rates fell long before vaccines."[26] Both experts present statistical information to support their conclusions. For many vaccine-preventable infections, the decrease in the number of reported cases, and/or the decrease in the severity of infections in Canada does appear to coincide with the approximate time period when the related vaccine was released. However, it is unclear whether this information is enough to conclude that vaccines make individuals healthier. The following is a discussion of why a closer look at how effective vaccines are at improving the health of a population is necessary:

- Historical epidemiological data is difficult to interpret. It is difficult to draw conclusions about the efficacy of vaccines based on incidence and death rates alone and without complete data or consideration of other factors that directly impact the health of a population, such as data limitations and public health improvements. Data limitations which can interfere with the assessment of the incidence and severity of infections over time include:

a. Inconsistent reporting over time, such as lack of data immediately prior to, or after the release of a vaccine; using different diagnostic criteria from one year to the next; and inconsistent reporting from one province or state to the next.
b. Lack of information about vaccination status, such as how many sick people were vaccinated and what percentage of the population was vaccinated.
c. Misdiagnosis of infections. For example, if a person was vaccinated against pertussis as a child and developed symptoms of pertussis as an adult, her doctor may wrongly assume that it is impossible for her to have contracted a pertussis infection due to her vaccination status, and thus may misdiagnose the infection.

Assessments regarding the role of vaccinations and their efficacy are difficult to make because many other factors can influence the health of a population and an individual's susceptibility to disease. Since the first vaccine for smallpox was invented at the turn of the eighteenth century, there have been many lifestyle and public health improvements that have undoubtedly contributed to improved health conditions over the years.

These advancements include the following:

a. Improved personal hygiene due to routine hand washing, indoor plumbing, filtered water, and organized sewage disposal.
b. Better nutrition through increased availability and diversity of food, education about healthy nutrition, and public awareness about sanitary food preparation.
c. Less exposure to infections through improved sanitation, refrigeration, safe farming practices, the isolation approach to infected persons, and public awareness about how infections spread.
d. Better health care due to improved health coverage, and improved methods of diagnosing and treating diseases.
e. Improved working and living conditions.

Other factors can have a negative impact on the health of a population by interfering with access to clean water, nutritious food, or medical care, and thus they increase the risk of a population's susceptibility to infections. These factors include:

a. Poverty and economic depressions, such as the Great Depression.
b. Large-scale wars, such as World War II.
c. Natural disasters such as earthquakes, floods, and storms as well as man-made disasters such as nuclear disasters.

d. High frequency of international travel to Third World countries.

All of these factors should be considered when drawing conclusions regarding the impact of public health initiatives on a population over time.

- Different strains of viruses and bacteria exist. Viruses and bacteria can undergo changes and create different strains (subtypes) with different characteristics. These changes can cause the virus and/or bacteria to be stronger or weaker. For example, there are over a hundred strains of the polio virus, but the most typical polio vaccine contains only three strains. If someone is exposed to a strain that he or she has not been vaccinated against, he or she may or may not be protected, depending on how closely the new strain resembles the one the individual was initially vaccinated against. Vaccines are typically created to protect against the most common or most severe strains of an infection, however, it is difficult to predict which strain an individual may be exposed to and how a virus or bacteria will change over time.

- Some vaccines have caused the infection they were meant to protect against. Live vaccines are used because they typically stimulate the immune system in a way that is more similar to a true infection than a dead vaccine, which results in better protection.[27] Although live vaccines contain weakened viruses or bacteria, they may still be able to cause infection if the immune system in question is in a susceptible state or if the weakened virus or bacteria mutates into a stronger form. For example, the live polio virus that is used in the oral polio vaccine (OPV) can revert to a stronger strain and cause paralytic polio.[28] The use of OPV in Canada has in fact caused cases of paralytic polio.[29] Eleven of the twelve cases of paralytic polio between 1980 and 1995 were caused by the oral polio vaccine.[30] Not only was the vaccine able to cause paralytic polio in vaccine recipients, but also in people who were in contact with people who received the vaccine (eight out of the eleven cases).[31] Paralytic polio resulting from vaccination is a recognized complication that can occur after vaccination for which the National Vaccine Compensation Program (US) offers compensation.[32] Although the live OPV has been largely replaced by the inactivated polio vaccine (IPV) in North America, the OPV is still used in many other countries.[33] Because of this risk, it is especially important for those whose immune systems are not functioning optimally or those who are currently battling another infection to consider the risks and benefits of live vaccines. Live vaccines commonly administered to children include measles, mumps, rubella, and varicella. More recently, the new AIDS vaccine, which was tested on people in Southern Africa, appears to make people more susceptible to being infected with HIV strains.[34]

- Some vaccines have failed to protect. There are many reports of outbreaks in vaccinated populations. In 2006, there were more than 2,500 cases of measles in the US and approximately half of the people affected had previously been vaccinated.[35] In 2002, there was a varicella outbreak in Minnesota where 59% of the children had been vaccinated against varicella.[36] The child who is assumed to have started the outbreak was vaccinated.[37] In this instance, there was a slight difference in the severity of varicella infection experienced by the vaccinated and unvaccinated group. Vaccinated students recovered one day faster than unvaccinated students. Vaccinated students were also less likely to have a fever and had fewer skin lesions, (children who were vaccinated had fewer than fifty skin lesions; children who were not had more than fifty).[38]

- Efficacy rates may not reflect the ability of a vaccine to protect against infection. Estimated efficacy rates for the vaccines commonly administered to Canadian children range from 70 to 100%.[39] Our perception of vaccine efficacy can easily be clouded due to miscommunication. Efficacy rates are, at times, based on the ability of people to generate a threshold number of antibodies in response to a vaccine, not the actual ability to fend off an infection. For example, the actual ability of the seasonal influenza vaccine to protect against infection in children aged six months to nineteen years ranges from 0 to 93%.[40] If the infecting influenza virus is similar to one of those found in the vaccine, the likelihood of protection is higher. However, the more dissimilar the infecting virus is from the one in the vaccine, the less protection the vaccine will offer. In fact, in children under two years, the inactivated seasonal influenza vaccine appears to be as effective as placebo and in healthy people under sixty-five vaccination does not appear to affect hospital stay, time off work, or death from influenza or its complications.[41] To add to the confusion, an individual could still be immune to an infection even if a blood test reveals that he or she does not have antibodies to an infection. Scientists and medical professionals are still trying to understand the intricacies of the immune system. More research and clarity is required to establish a realistic expectation of short- and long-term vaccine efficacy.

- Vaccine-induced immunity can wear off. A number of studies reveal a trend of decreased efficacy of vaccine-induced immunity over time.[42,43,44] For example, the efficacy of a meningococcal vaccine was evaluated one year after injection in the UK. After only twelve months, vaccinated infants had no demonstrable protection against meningitis and the efficacy in toddlers decreased from 88% to 61%.[45] Younger vaccine recipients typically require more vaccine boosters than adults in order to maintain an adequate number of antibodies after vaccination.[46] Some vaccines are believed to provide lifelong protection against infection[47] (e.g., polio); others are thought to confer a shorter term of protection (e.g., diphtheria and tetanus) and therefore require regular boosters.[48] There are also vaccines which only protect for a very short time (e.g., flu).[49] The degree of protection that is provided after vaccination appears to vary with the vaccine and the recipient. By contrast, natural immunity obtained from naturally acquired infections often provides lifelong immunity because the immunized person can overcome the initial infection.

Another issue associated with waning efficacy is that females who are vaccinated as children may have lost their immunity before they become pregnant. If, for example, a woman becomes infected with measles, rubella, varicella, or hepatitis B during pregnancy, she has an increased risk of miscarriage and/or giving birth to a baby with birth defects. This is also true for a number of other infections that are not vaccinated against. It is likely that more and more recommendations for booster vaccines in adolescents and adults will occur in order to compensate for the loss of immunity over time. Mothers who have naturally acquired immunity to an infection, pass on antibodies to their unborn child through the placenta and also through breast milk. If a mother's immunity has worn off for a specific infection, she will not pass on protective antibodies for that infection to her child, which results in infants being more susceptible to infections in the first year of life (as seen with the use of the measles vaccine).[50]

- Vaccines can shift infections to target younger and older populations. Children who are vaccinated may escape infection at a young age, but waning immunity means that, with time, they can once again become susceptible. One example is the increasing incidence of pertussis in adolescents and adults[51] which followed the decreasing incidence of pertussis in children. This trend may also be seen with other infections where vaccines do not provide long-term immunity and is a concern because infections that are usually mild in childhood may affect people more severely as they age. In addition, the symptoms in children may be different than those present in adolescents and adults, which may lead to delays in diagnosis and treatment.

- Some vaccines may contribute to diseases and infections. The most notorious example of a vaccine-induced infection is the introduction of *simian virus 40* into humans through the oral and injected polio vaccines in the US and Canada in the 1950s and 1960s.[52] (Refer to chapter 3, "Specific Vaccination Issues," for further details). *The Virus and The Vaccine: Contaminated Vaccine, Deadly Cancers and Government Neglect*, is a book by investigative journalists Debbie Bookchin and Jim Schumacher which examines these events in greater detail. Dr. Leonard Horowitz has written a book, which argues that the AIDS virus (HIV) was also introduced into humans by contaminated vaccines.[53] There is a very slight possibility that Creutzfeldt-Jacob Disease (CJD), a very serious brain disease with no known cure,[54] can result from vaccines if they are accidentally made using contaminated cow products (more information on CJD in the immune system section of chapter 3).

  Macrophagic myofasciitis (MMF) is a newly identified disease that appears to be associated with vaccines that contain aluminum.[55] MMF is characterized by muscle aches, joint aches, and chronic fatigue.[56] The onset of MMF can occur within months to years after vaccination.[57] Joint pain, muscle aches, and fatigue are commonly reported post-vaccination symptoms[58] and, interestingly, these symptoms are also very often reported in clinical practice. Therefore, there may be many more cases of MMF than have been diagnosed. Vaccines have also been implicated in immune system disorders (see the immune system section in chapter 3 for details). Preliminary research suggests that people who previously received the seasonal influenza vaccine may be at a higher risk of contracting the pandemic influenza H1N1.[59] Due to the limitations in vaccine monitoring, conditions that are triggered by vaccination but diagnosed months to years after vaccination are likely not currently associated with vaccines.

- Vaccines are sensitive. Vaccines are sensitive to excessive changes in temperature. There is some concern that the improper transportation and storage of vaccines can lead to the decreased efficacy of these products.[60]

- The health of the person also plays a role. Modern medicine has focused much of its efforts on isolating and identifying infectious agents such as viruses and bacteria. While this focus has been helpful in developing specific medical treatments for infections, the role of the health of the individual is often overlooked. Some people may get the flu three times over the span of three months, while others who are exposed to the flu virus show no flu-like symptoms at all. Though it is rare, people may die from complications of the flu, as is true of many other infections. After being exposed to an infection, one person may be asymptomatic, while another person may have a mild infection and recover quickly, and still another individual may have a long-lasting illness with severe complications. The reasons for these differences is unclear. Much more effort should be placed on understanding how an individual's current health status impacts his/her susceptibility to infectious diseases. Many factors can affect our immune system such as stress level, nutritional status and toxic load. Consequently, there are many steps we can take to help our children stay healthy. For more information, see the accompanying workbook *Childhood Vaccinations: Making Informed Decisions*.

## *What about herd immunity?*

Herd immunity is the concept that if most people are immune to an infection, the infection will not be able to spread throughout the population. For example, if one person falls ill and that person is surrounded by a community of people who are already immune to the infection, the infection cannot spread to the general population. The benefit of herd immunity is that the herd can act as a buffer, and protect a few more vulnerable people who are not yet immune to that infection. Some people cannot be vaccinated because they have an immune condition that would put them at a high risk of a complication from a vaccine and many others cannot be vaccinated because they are pregnant. If the majority of people in the herd have already developed immunity to an infection (either naturally or through a vaccine) the more susceptible individuals may be protected from being exposed to that infection. However, it is difficult to establish and maintain herd immunity in our modern world because international travel is commonplace and there are no international standards on vaccination. Also, vaccination does not guarantee immunity and vaccine-induced immunity can wear off with time and leave people once again susceptible to infection. In the case of common and mild childhood infections, there may be a reduced number of people who develop life long immunity through mass vaccination strategies, which, in fact, decreases our population's natural herd immunity over time.

For example, before the varicella vaccine, 90% of children were naturally exposed to the varicella virus by the time they reached twelve years of age.[61] Now that this vaccine is part of the recommended childhood vaccination schedule, the percentage of children who will be exposed to the natural varicella virus will likely decrease. If the varicella vaccine does not provide lifelong immunity, vaccinated children will grow into susceptible adolescents and adults. Adults and adolescents are at a higher risk of complications including pneumonia, encephalitis, and death.[62] Varicella can also be dangerous to an unborn child if a woman is infected during pregnancy.[63] Measles, mumps, and rubella are other infections, which are considered to be milder if an individual is exposed during childhood. As well, an exposure to these infections usually results in an individual's lifelong immunity.[64] Some parents even consider the benefit of intentionally allowing their child to be exposed to some of the milder infections in order to increase the likelihood that they will develop lifelong immunity.

Here are some other thoughts to consider when weighing the benefits and risks of vaccinating for the benefit of the community:

- Following the recommended vaccination schedule may provide protection against fewer than twenty infections for an undetermined amount of time. The groups most susceptible to complications from infections are typically those who are very young, very old, people with a compromised immune system, and pregnant women. There are many people who fall into these categories and there are many other infections that could be dangerous to them, besides infections targeted by vaccines.
- A few of the vaccines that we use are live, in other words, they contain an infectious agent that is still active. A live vaccine may infrequently cause the infection it was meant to protect against. In addition, there is a very slight risk that a vaccine may be contaminated with another infectious agent (see the immune system section in chapter 3 for details). Infections inadvertently caused by a vaccine could spread to others.
- It is difficult to predict the impact of mass vaccinations on the overall health of a population because we have not yet assessed the long-term health risks of vaccinating. Vaccines may be decreasing the incidence or severity of some infections, but whether they improve the overall health of our population is as yet unclear. Likewise, it is difficult to predict the impact of mass vaccinations on

the health of future generations. Modern science is only starting to understand our interdependence with viruses, bacteria, and parasites. The medical community knows that bacteria constitute a large part of our biological makeup. In fact, an adult human contains ten times as many microbial cells as it does human cells.[65] As well, recent discoveries indicate that viral and bacterial DNA sequences are found in our DNA.[66] Recent research is also uncovering the ways in which bacteria and parasites actually help us stay healthy and how other microbes may influence human behaviour.[67] In addition, there is rising concern that serious infections that we eradicate through vaccinations could be used as biochemical warfare.[68] For example, since we have eradicated smallpox worldwide, we no longer vaccinate against smallpox. Our population could once again be exposed to smallpox as some laboratories still contain live smallpox viruses. There are some who speculate that the smallpox virus has not been completely annihilated, but that mutations have disguised it as a different infection (e.g., monkey pox). We cannot be completely confident that our vaccination strategies have ensured the safety of our population, as well as future generations.

There are many factors that can affect a person's health. Making a conscious effort to keep your family physically, mentally, emotionally, and spiritually healthy will positively impact the people around you. In addition, encouraging only "healthy" play dates and keeping sick children at home and away from susceptible individuals is recommended.

## *Does vaccination pose ethical questions?*

There are a variety of ethical conflicts regarding the delivery of childhood vaccinations to the public. The following is a discussion of some of the major ethical issues.

- The lack of clear information regarding the benefits and risks of each vaccination option. Parents who question and express concern regarding the risks associated with vaccines are frequently given the explanation that "the benefits far outweigh the risks." This blanket response is not helpful for parents who want to understand the benefits and risks of vaccinating their child. This statement is also inaccurate since the medical community does not currently have a true estimate of the risks involved (see the sections on risks of vaccines and safety in this chapter for discussion). Very few people are presented with the information they require to make an informed decision. Health care providers should help parents understand the benefits and risks of all options available to them.

- Lack of independent vaccine safety evaluation. Please see the previous discussion in the safety section of this chapter.

- Revenue from vaccines may influence the clinical use of vaccines. Vaccines are a multibillion dollar per year business. For example, the Canadian government spent approximately $225 million on vaccines in one year (2001/2002).[69] One prominent American vaccine manufacturer declared sales of over one billion dollars worth of vaccines in one year (2005).[70] Making money from the sale of vaccines is not in itself an ethical conflict, but the influence of such a large industry on medical education, scientific research, and clinical practice is worth considering. In a recent interview Dr. Stephen Choi, the former editor-in-chief of the Canadian Medical Association Journal (CMAJ),[71] said that "most medical journals are funded by the drug industry by way of advertisement" and that "it doesn't take much to realize the potential for conflict of interest exists."[72] Dr. Choi and a number of former CMAJ editors and board members have recently launched their own independent peer-reviewed medical journal in response to an incident where "information and debate have been stifled because of private and political concerns of making knowledge public."[73] Their new journal, *Open Medicine*, does not accept advertising from the pharmaceutical industry and is available online at www.openmedicine.ca. There are already a few articles published by this journal that discuss the conflicts of interest that exist regarding the role of the pharmaceutical industry in the practice of medicine. There are also a number of books written by medical doctors that address the pharmaceutical industry's influence on medical education and practice, which include the following:

a. *Powerful Medicines: The Benefits, Risks, and Costs of Prescription Drugs* by Dr. Jerry Avorn MD

b. *Overdosed America: The Broken Promise of American Medicine* by Dr. John Abramson MD
c. *The Truth About the Drug Companies: How They Deceive Us and What to Do About It* by Dr. Marcia Angell MD
d. *The Medical Mafia: How to Get Out Of It Alive and Take Back our Health and Wealth* by Dr. Guylaine Lanctot

- Vaccination is often mandatory or perceived to be mandatory. Every year, undervaccinated Canadian children are sent home from school and are not welcome back until they have proof that their vaccines are up to date. No other option is offered. As a result, most Canadian parents are under the impression that in order for their child to attend daycare and school, they must be fully vaccinated. Some have also been informed by their child's pediatrician that if they refuse the recommended vaccines, their child will no longer be treated at that clinic. Even though childhood vaccines are not mandatory in Canada, most parents perceive them to be. In other areas vaccines may be truly mandatory and a parent may be threatened with incarceration, financial penalty, or removal of the child from the parent's care. In light of the lack of clear and objective vaccine safety and efficacy information available, the ethical dilemma is whether parents or the government is best suited to make vaccination decisions for children.

- Lack of compensation for people who have been injured by vaccines. If people were well aware of the risks and their options regarding childhood vaccinations, the lack of compensation would not be considered an ethical conflict because people would then be consciously making a choice to undertake a risk. This is not the case for most Canadians who are not aware of the possible risks and believe that childhood vaccines are mandatory. In Canada, only Quebec has a legal process in place to provide compensation to vaccine-injured families. Quebec's "no fault" vaccination compensation system[74] is similar to the National Vaccine Injury Compensation Program (VICP)[75] in the US. Since the VICP program began in 1998, it has paid out over 700 million dollars to families affected by complications due to vaccinations.[76] These compensation programs are far from ideal as many families are not able to prove that the injury or death following vaccination was solely due to the vaccine, especially if limited funds are available or if the complication did not occur immediately following the administration of the vaccine. In addition, a "no fault" system means that no one is held accountable, therefore, there is less motivation for manufacturers to continually improve vaccine safety.

Chapter 3

# SPECIFIC VACCINATION ISSUES

Do vaccines harm the immune system?

Do vaccines cause autism?

Do vaccines cause sudden infant death syndrome?

Should I worry about mercury in vaccines?

## Key Concepts

*Vaccines may contribute to some immune system disorders.*

*Vaccines may contribute to some cases of autism and other neurological disorders.*

*Vaccines may contribute to some cases of sudden infant death.*

*The mercury and aluminum found in some vaccines is of concern.*

## SPECIFIC VACCINATION ISSUES

Note: This chapter includes information about controversial vaccine issues that require more scientific research and the level of detail may be overwhelming for some readers. For some parents, awareness of these issues and the strong recommendation of further research is sufficient. Others may be eager to understand the controversy and read the details, which is why they are included in this chapter.

### *Do vaccines harm the immune system?*

It is often said that vaccines help to strengthen our immune systems, but it is unclear how this is measured. Antibodies are frequently created after a vaccine is injected, but this is not enough to conclude that our immune systems are more robust after vaccination.

Despite these claims developed countries such as Canada and the US have seen a recent increase in immune system disorders and inflammatory conditions such as allergies,[1] asthma,[2] arthritis,[3] as well as autoimmune conditions, such as multiple sclerosis[4] and juvenile type 1 diabetes.[5] In fact, Canada has one of the highest incidences of multiple sclerosis in the world,[6] and as many as one in ten North Americans are affected by autoimmune diseases.[7]

Establishing a vaccine as the only cause of an immune disorder is very difficult as the symptoms of these conditions may not surface immediately after the injection of a vaccine. Inflammatory and autoimmune diseases may need to progress to the point of tissue destruction before symptoms are noticed and this detection may take months or years. There are also other factors that may contribute to the development of abnormal immune function, including the following:

- A highly sanitary lifestyle may interfere with proper immune system development.[8] Early childhood infections appear to be necessary to promote optimal functioning of the immune system.
- Increased exposures to environmental toxins can interfere with optimal immune system function. Infants are much more susceptible to the negative effects of toxins than adults. New research suggests that exposure to toxins in utero could result in adult onset disorders in not only the first generation, but subsequent generations as well.[9]
- A poor diet and prolonged psychological stress can interfere with the function of all body systems (including the immune system).

- Modifications in diagnostic criteria required to diagnose immune system disorders can affect statistics from one year to another.

It is likely that more than one factor is contributing to the rise of immune disorders. However, there is evidence to show that vaccines may play a role in interfering with proper immune system development and function. Below are some of the current concerns regarding the effect of vaccines on the immune system. The information below outlines why additional resources and research are needed to understand the long-term effects of vaccines on the immune system:

- Vaccines may interfere with proper immune system development.

    a. Vaccines can disrupt immune cell balance. Vaccines have been implicated as a causative factor or trigger in various immune system disorders including allergic conditions (e.g., asthma,[10] allergies,[11] arthritis,[12] and atopic dermatitis,[13]), as well as autoimmune diseases (e.g., arthritis,[14,15] lupus,[16] diabetes mellitus type 1,[17] thrombocytopenia,[18] polymyositis/dermatomyositis,[19] polyarteritis nodosa,[20] Bell's palsy,[21] and Guillain Barré syndrome).[22] Vaccines can cause a relative predominance of either T-helper 1 (Th1) or T-helper 2 (Th2) immune cells.[23,24] T helper cells are immune cells that play an important role in activating and communicating with other components of the immune system. Infant immune systems begin with a relative predominance of Th2 cells.[25] With exposure to infections, infants gradually develop a Th1/Th2 balance.[26] It is normal for either Th1 or Th2 cells to predominate at different times; however, problems arise when either Th1 or Th2 cells predominate for prolonged periods of time.[27] Chronic Th1 cell predominance is seen in some autoimmune associated diseases (e.g., Hashimoto's thyroiditis, multiple sclerosis, type 1 diabetes mellitus, and Crohns' disease), whereas chronic Th2 cell predominance is seen in some inflammatory conditions (e.g., asthma, eczema, and allergies), as well as cancer, chronic fatigue, immune deficiency syndrome, and other diseases.[28] Vaccines that interfere with the Th1/Th2 balance may contribute to the development of immune disorders.

b. Injected vaccines bypass the external immune system. Human beings come into contact with many different types of bacteria and viruses every day without being aware of it. Most of these bacteria and viruses do not enter our bodies because humans have evolved a sophisticated immune system. One key component of the immune system is located on the outside of our bodies and is called mucosal immunity. It is the first line of defence of the immune system. A mucous membrane is the moist skin that lines openings of the body such as the inside of the nose and the mouth. Most infections enter the body through mucous membranes. Mucous membranes are coated with protective antibodies, enzymes, and secretions that prevent bacteria and viruses from binding to and entering the body. Mucosal immunity is not well understood at this time.[29] Components of the outer immune system communicate with the inner immune system. The injection of vaccines introduces antigens directly into our bodies and thus bypasses the first line of defence. Once inside the body, antigens can enter the bloodstream more easily and become distributed to the rest of the body. Vaccination is very different from what happens during a natural infection. A natural infection usually results from a virus or bacteria first crossing through the mucous membrane,[30] which stimulates events within the inner immune system. There is some concern that in susceptible individuals the immune system may respond to this "surprise attack" by overreacting which leads to inflammatory conditions. The immune system may also become hypersensitive, which leads to autoimmune diseases. There is not yet a clear understanding of the long-term health impact of bypassing the first line of defence by injecting developing infants with vaccines. In addition to potentially disrupting the immune system, there is some evidence to show that injected vaccines may not be the best protection against infections. Infections that pass through the mucous membrane stimulate the immune system to create antibodies and place them in the location where the infection entered the body. Injected vaccines result in the concentration of protective antibodies and immune cells inside the body. The benefit of having antibodies on the exterior of the body (coating the mucous membranes) is that they are able to prevent viruses and bacteria from binding to and entering the body.[31,32] For example, the oral polio vaccine, which is taken by mouth, is better able to stimulate the production of protective antibodies on mucous membranes than the injected polio vaccine.[33]

c. Injection of multiple vaccines may overburden the immune system. The recommended vaccination schedule in Canada begins with four injections (although the provincial guidelines vary). These four injections include a total of sixteen different strains of viruses and bacteria (refer to Figure 4), which means that an infant's immune system is challenged to respond to sixteen different antigens simultaneously at two months of age. Infants are, of course, exposed to viruses and bacteria on a daily basis. In fact, the development of the immune system is thought to partially rely on this "immune system training.'" However, few infections are able to move past the first line of immune defence and enter the body at one time. With vaccines, antigens are directly injected into the body all at once while bypassing the mucosal immunity. The Institute of Medicine (IOM), a non-profit organization in the US, which strives to provide unbiased and evidence-based information and advice regarding health and science policy, recently reviewed the issue of overburdening infants' immune systems and concluded that infants' immune systems are capable of responding to many different antigens and infections at one time. Despite the IOM's findings, there is still some concern that an immature immune system may be overwhelmed from having to work so hard at a very young age, especially when antigens are introduced in an unnatural way and in combination with a variety of chemicals which can negatively impact the immune system.

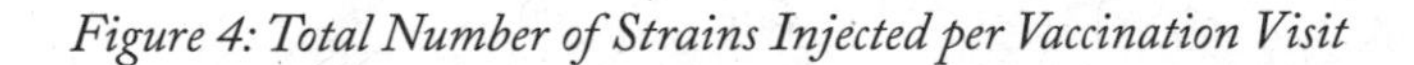

*Figure 4: Total Number of Strains Injected per Vaccination Visit*

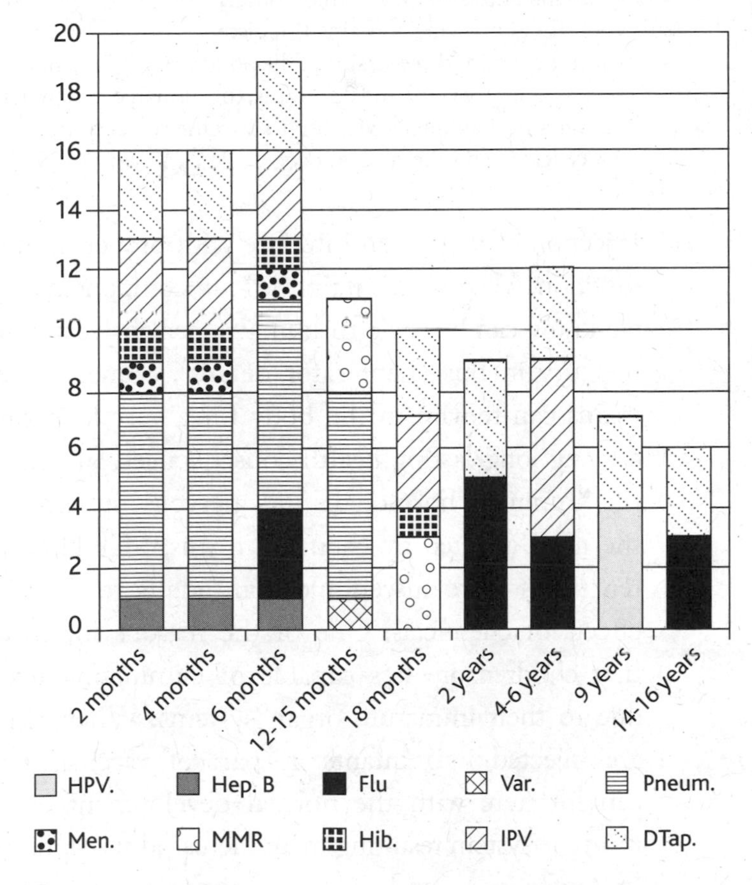

*Notes about the data:*

- Source: The schedule used is the national recommended vaccination schedule for Canadian Children in 2009.[34] The number of different types of strains in each vaccine is from the Public Health Agency of Canada.[35]
- The US schedule includes vaccines against two additional types of infections, which are not included in Figure 4.
- The flu vaccine is recommended once per year starting at 6 months and three doses of HPV are required. These are not included in Figure 4.
- Some vaccines contain more than one bacterial or viral strain (subtype). The flu vaccine contains three strains of the flu virus, the polio vaccine contains three strains of the polio virus,[36] pneumococcal vaccines contain between 7 and 23 strains, the human papillomavirus vaccine contains 4 strains.[37] Meningitis vaccine refers to the single meningococcal C and the meningococcal A, C, Y and W135.

d. Injection of toxins can interfere with proper immune function. Vaccines contain various components that we know can be toxic to humans (see the section on mercury in this chapter for details). Some of these toxins can remain in the body for a very long time, causing long-lasting health consequences. In general, the immune, hormonal, and nervous systems are the most affected by chemical toxins.[38] Children are ten times more susceptible than adults to the toxic effects of chemicals. One of the reasons for this is that children are less capable of eliminating toxins due to their immature organ systems. When toxins are injected into infants as part of vaccines, they can interfere with the normal development of the immune system resulting in an increased susceptibility to infections and chronic immune disorders.

e. Pain from repeated injections may affect future immunity. Local pain is a common side effect from vaccines. A recent animal study revealed that early pain experiences in newborns can adversely affect the infant's health long term, and may include effects such as long-lasting hypersensitivity to pain and a decreased immune response.[39] Other common post-natal procedures that can be painful include vitamin K injections, blood tests, eye antibiotics, and circumcision. The recommended vaccination schedule in Canada includes fourteen injections within the first year. Although all painful experiences for newborns cannot be eliminated, these surprising findings warrant more investigation due to the potential long-term health effects.

- Vaccines can cause infections

a. Live vaccines can cause the infections they were meant to protect against. Paralytic polio and measles are known potential side effects of live polio and measles vaccines. Live vaccines introduce a weakened virus or bacteria, which can cause an acute infection if the strain mutates into a stronger virus or bacteria, or if the person's immune system is compromised and not able to combat even weak infections. Mild, persistent vaccine-induced infections may also have a negative impact on overall health. For example, persistent vaccine-induced measles infection in the digestive system may be linked to some forms of autism, (see the autism section in this chapter for details).

b. Vaccines can be contaminated with other infectious agents. Some vaccines may be contaminated with viruses and bacteria or other infectious agents that are unintentionally included in the vaccine. The contamination of polio vaccines (oral and injected forms) with a monkey virus SV40 in North America between 1955 and 1963 is well documented.[40] This occurred because the vaccine's active ingredient was grown in monkey kidney cells.[41,42] The long-term impact of having injected humans with this monkey virus is unclear, but there is some concern that the SV40 virus has had a role in the development of some cancers. Studies show that the SV40 virus has the ability to transform healthy human cells into cancerous cells and the virus has been found in various human cancerous tumours, (e.g., non-Hodgkin's lymphomas, osteosarcomas, mesotheliomas, and ependymomas).[43] SV40 also contaminated two other types of vaccines during the same time period.[44] It is unclear if the monkey virus was able to be transmitted from people who contracted the SV40 virus through a vaccine to other people who were not vaccinated.[45] Therefore, even those who were not vaccinated may have been affected by the introduction of a new virus into humans. Some speculate that HIV (human immunodeficiency virus) originated from vaccines contaminated with the monkey virus SIV (simian immunodeficiency virus).[46,47]

c. Manufacturers undertake various efforts to ensure that only the intended viruses and bacteria are included in vaccines. However, recent discoveries of other infectious agents such as prions (infectious proteins) and nanobacteria (very small bacteria) raise questions about the ability to screen for every infectious agent and release "pure" vaccines. Little is known about prions and their effect on health. Creutzfeldt-Jakob disease (CJD) is a serious infection believed to be caused by prions.[48] CJD is the human variant of bovine spongiform encephalopathy,[49] or mad cow disease. In 2005, there were twenty-three reported cases of CJD in Canada.[50] There are an average of 200 cases in the US per year.[51] The international incidence rate is approximately one case per one million.[52] CJD is a progressive neurological disease that is usually lethal within months.[53] There is no treatment available and the medical community is unsure whether prions can be transmitted through casual contact.[54] CJD is believed to be contracted through eating contaminated beef products; however, some vaccines are also made using cow products. The estimated risk of contracting CJD from vaccines that are made using cow materials is very low.[55,56] However, the fact that there is a risk suggests that there could be other unidentified infectious agents that are distributed through contaminated vaccines.

## *Do vaccines cause autism?*

Many parents and health care professionals are concerned about the vaccine–autism connection and some believe that the recent increase in reported cases of autism and other neurological disorders (e.g., learning disorders) is associated with vaccines. Autism may be caused by a variety of factors such as exposure to environmental toxins and viruses, unidentified sensitivities to gluten (found in wheat and other grains) or casein (found in dairy), digestive system disorders and genetics.[57] Understandably, vaccines have been under scrutiny because they are typically administered throughout childhood and can expose children to environmental toxins and viruses. Autism may develop gradually and symptoms may not appear immediately after injection. This makes it particularly difficult to identify a vaccine as a trigger. The first study that linked vaccines to autism was published in 1998 by Canadian-trained gastroenterologist Dr. Andrew Wakefield and eleven others.[58] As with other researchers who have published findings that question the safety of vaccines, Dr. Wakefield's research and scientific integrity have been severely scrutinized and the original article was eventually retracted in 2010. In 2004, the Institute of Medicine (IOM) reviewed a number of studies and concluded that there is no connection between the measles-mumps-rubella vaccine (MMR) and autism.[59] The IOM's report, however, also states that its findings do not exclude the possibility that the MMR vaccine contributes to autism in a small number of children.[60] In addition, the possible connection between autism and the combined administration of all the recommended vaccines has not yet been investigated. Unfortunately, despite these shortcomings, the IOM's report has put the vaccine–autism issue to rest for many parents and physicians. It is likely that most parents have seen a news or journal article that states that there is "no evidence that vaccines cause...autism,"[61] however, there is evidence to show that some cases of autism may be due to vaccines. Below is a discussion of why it is imperative that the possible vaccine–autism link be examined.

- Reports of regressive autism following administration of a live virus vaccine. A significant number of parents have reported that their child's symptoms of autism began after they received the MMR vaccine.[62,63] The subtype of autism that may be associated with the measles–mumps–rubella vaccine is regressive autism,[64] which accounts for up to 40% of cases of autism. Children diagnosed with regressive autism may appear normal for the first year or so, then begin to regress through developmental milestones such as loss of speech and motor abilities previously achieved. However, the symptoms are not limited to behavioural symptoms as described in classical autism cases.[65] Children diagnosed with regressive autism commonly have symptoms of excessive thirst, bowel disturbances, self-injury, cravings for particular foods, inflammatory skin conditions, and recurrent respiratory infections.[66] Some children with regressive autism have a persistent measles infection in their digestive tract, which may be caused by the live measles vaccine. This persistent infection may be enough to cause severe disturbances in the digestive, immune, and neurological systems. There may also be some connection between the use of antibiotics (which can also be found in some MMR vaccines) and the onset of regressive autistic symptoms.[67]

- Some causes of autism may be due to vaccines that contain mercury or other neurotoxins. The Vaccine Safety Datalink (VSD) is a large database that includes detailed vaccine reports and medical histories of millions of Americans. Two independent researchers, both medical doctors, were permitted to view the raw data in the VSD. The father-and-son team Geier and Geier have published in prestigious medical journals such as the *Journal of American Physicians and Surgeons* and concluded that thimerosal-containing vaccines result in a significantly increased risk of autism and other neurological disorders compared to thimerosal-free vaccines.[68] These findings are a concern since some of the vaccines that are used for pregnant women still contain thimerosal, which is roughly 50% mercury, and mercury readily passes through the placenta and breast milk. Although most of the mercury has been removed from childhood vaccines, children may still be exposed to mercury through vaccines (see the mercury section later in this chapter for more information). Too much mercury can cause spasms, tingling, numbness, irritability, restlessness, difficulty concentrating, decreased memory, depression, unsteady balance, speech disturbances, and tremors.[69] Many of these symptoms resemble those found in autistic children.[70] Therefore, some cases of autism may actually be misdiagnosed cases of mercury toxicity,[71] especially in children who received vaccines prior to the mid-1990s (when much more mercury was added to children's vaccines). Children who have already been exposed to mercury through other sources or who have a health condition that would make them more susceptible to the toxic effects of mercury are at higher risk of mercury toxicity. The good news is that neurological symptoms often improve with the removal of mercury from the body.[72,73,74] It is likely that some children are more susceptible to mercury and other neurotoxins. This may be because they have difficulty removing toxins from their body or because they have already been exposed to toxins and their cumulative dose is higher than average. More research is required before we can conclude that vaccines that contain heavy metals and other potential neurotoxins are not interfering with the normal development of the infant neurological system.

- Reports of complications caused by vaccines include a wide variety of neurological symptoms. Reported complications from vaccinations in Canada in 2004 include numbness, paralysis, convulsions, unresponsiveness, extreme sleepiness, loss of muscle tone, abnormally slow or few body movements, Guillain Barré syndrome, and other symptoms of nervous system dysfunction.[75] These complications suggest that vaccines can have a variety of negative effects on the nervous system in some people. Some neurological conditions may not yet be associated with vaccines, especially if the onset is not apparent immediately after vaccination.

- Vaccines may cause autism by instigating an abnormal immune reaction. As previously discussed in the immune system section of this chapter, vaccines may be the cause of some immune system disorders. Autism may be triggered by an autoimmune reaction[76] or another type of abnormal immune function[77] following vaccination. Dr. Andrew Moulden is a controversial Canadian medical doctor and neuroscientist who has concluded that all vaccines can cause an immune reaction that results in microvascular strokes (small disruptions of blood flow). According to Dr. Moulden, evidence of these ministrokes can appear within five days of vaccination and these ministrokes cause tissue damage, which, Moulden suspects, is the cause of a wide variety of chronic illnesses and disorders including autism. For more information about his findings, visit http://brainguardmd.com.

## *Do vaccines cause sudden infant death syndrome?*

The diagnosis of sudden infant death syndrome (SIDS) is given to a previously healthy child under the age of one year who has died suddenly due to an unknown cause (e.g., not due to choking, suffocation, or abuse).[78] An autopsy and post-mortem testing is required for this diagnosis. SIDS rates in Canada and the US have been progressively decreasing since 1990.[79,80] This decline is likely due to the public awareness campaigns, which include suggestions such as placing infants to sleep on their backs on a firm surface in a smoke-free environment and taking steps to ensure that infants are not overheating. For more information regarding risk factors of SIDS, consult the National Sudden and Unexplained Infant/Child Pregnancy Loss Resource Center (www.sidscenter.org) or the Canadian Foundation for the Study of Infant Deaths (www.sidscanada.org). Every year, however, many babies in developed countries still die suddenly from unidentified causes. SIDS is the leading cause of death in infants one month to one year old in the US.[81] There were 62 cases of SIDS in Canada and an additional 35 cases diagnosed as sudden unexplained deaths in 2003.[82] Sudden unexplained death is the diagnosis used for sudden infant deaths that do not fit the SIDS criteria. In 2003, the IOM reviewed a number of studies and concluded that SIDS is not caused by injections that contain multiple vaccines,[83] but the IOM also stated that there is insufficient information to determine whether multiple vaccines cause sudden unexplained death in infancy[84] or whether vaccines for hepatitis B, *Haemophilus influenzae* type b, polio, or the vaccine for diphtheria, tetanus and pertussis increase the risk of SIDS.[85]

It is therefore too early to draw the conclusion that "vaccines do not cause SIDS."[86] Vaccines have caused deaths in Canadian children and there is insufficient information regarding the role of vaccines in sudden infant deaths. A thorough vaccine surveillance system, complete post-mortem testing, and appropriate long-term research is required before conclusions can be drawn.

Below is some information that reinforces why it is important that we continue to investigate the possible connection between vaccines and sudden infant deaths, (including SIDS and other sudden deaths).

- Deaths closely following vaccinations. SIDS is a rare occurrence for infants under one month of age[87] and it is most commonly seen when infants reach two to four months,[88] which is when most infants in North America receive their first two doses of vaccines. Reports of deaths following vaccine administration are rare; however, it is unknown how many deaths following vaccinations are not reported as a possible vaccine complication. As mentioned in chapter 2, there were eight reports filed of deaths following vaccinations in Canada between 1992–2004.[89] These reports were reviewed and three of the eight deaths were later attributed to an administered vaccine.[90] In each of the three deaths, the tuberculosis vaccine was implicated.[91] This vaccine is not typically part of the standard recommended children's vaccines.

  Ninety-nine reports of deaths were submitted to the VAERS database following vaccination in US children aged 0 to 17 years in 2008.[92] Some of the deaths occurred within hours of vaccine administration in previously healthy children. The majority of child deaths reported occurred within one week of vaccine administration (see Figure 5) and in children under six months of age.

*Figure 5: Reported Deaths Following Vaccination in US Children Aged 0–17 Years in 2008.*

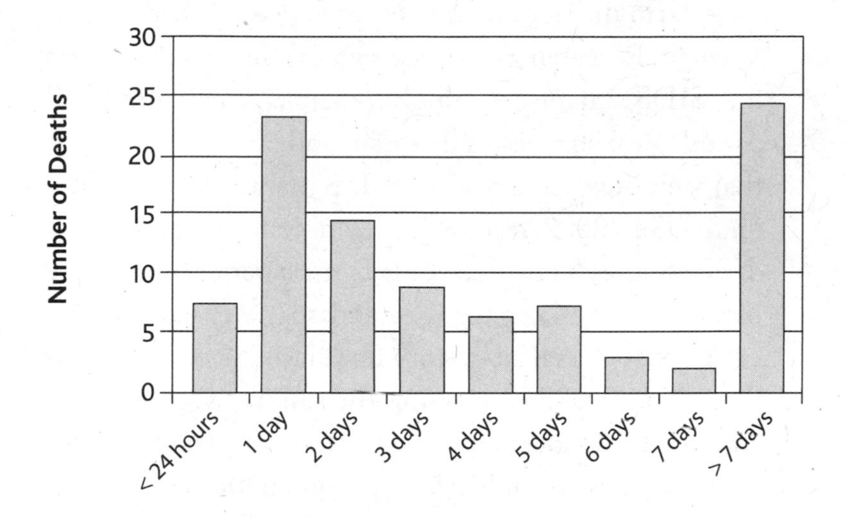


*Notes about the data:*

- Source of data: US Government's VAERS Database.[93]
- A report filed does not mean that a vaccine was determined as the cause of the adverse event.
- Five reports of deaths in US children in 2008 following vaccination did not have an associated timeline and have been omitted from figure 5.
- Since it is estimated that only 0 to 13% of serious adverse events to drugs are reported in the US,[94] the numbers above likely represent a very small portion of the total number of true adverse events.
- For additional limitations on data, consult VAERS.[95]

- Flaws in post-mortem testing. Many of the VAERS reports indicate the cause of death to be sudden unexplained death or sudden infant death syndrome. The diagnosis of SIDS requires an autopsy, an investigation of the circumstances of death, and a medical history.[96] If it is unclear what has caused these deaths, the assumption cannot be made that the injection of modified viruses, bacteria, and toxins into infants is not a contributing factor. It is important to perform the right tests in order to determine the cause of death. Researchers in Italy suggest that standard tests for SIDS infants overlook possible vaccine-induced pathological changes in the brain and heart.[97] Guidelines that were suggested at the 7th International Conference on SIDS in 2002, recommend a more thorough autopsy of SIDS cases "performed only by an experienced, reliable pathologist."[98] Diagnostic standards are essential to ensure that crucial laboratory findings are not omitted as they could establish or refute the link between vaccines and SIDS. Inadequate diagnostic measures may also cloud our understanding of another condition that may be associated with vaccinations: shaken baby syndrome.

- Misdiagnosis of shaken baby syndrome cases. Many cases of shaken baby syndrome (SBS) do not have visible signs of trauma.[99] Even though child abuse without blatant external signs of trauma undoubtedly does occur, it is possible that some children who have been diagnosed with SBS have a different underlying cause. Dr. Alan Clemetson was a researcher, medical professor, and medical doctor who was suspicious of the origin of the diagnostic criteria for SBS because of the significant overlap between the symptoms of SBS and acute vitamin C deficiency.[100] Both share symptoms of bruising, fractures of ribs and the ends of long bones, bleeding in and around the brain, and bleeding in the retina of the eye.[101] Acute vitamin C deficiency may be brought on by vaccination in a person whose vitamin C status is already depleted,[102] but vitamin C deficiency is often overlooked. Because of the overlap in symptoms, some cases of acute vitamin C deficiency may be misdiagnosed as SBS. Dr. Archie Kalokerinos is a researcher, medical doctor, and author of the book *Every Second Child*. Dr. Kalokerinos has observed that an alarming number of children under his care died after the administration of the diphtheria-tetanus-pertussis vaccine[103] and he was able to greatly reduce the number of deaths by administering vitamin C before, with, or after vaccination.[104] The incidence of SBS in Canada and the US peaks at two to four months, the time period when the first two sets of vaccines are commonly administered. In Japan, the peak incidence period is seven to nine months and corresponds to their initial set of vaccinations.[105] Since the incidence of SBS is estimated to be quite high (the very conservative estimate is of 40 cases per year in Canada, 25 cases per 100,000 children under one year in the US and the United Kingdom[106]), it seems appropriate to add vitamin C status as part of the diagnostic tests when evaluating some cases of SBS.

- Sudden death due to stress. Canadian epidemiologist Dr. Hans Selye spent many years researching the effects of stress on the body. He concluded that viruses, bacteria, and toxins (among other factors), can act as stressors on the body. He states that if stress overwhelms the body, death can ensue immediately or within days.[107] All three of these stressors – viruses, bacteria, and toxins – are found in vaccines. Dr. Viera Scheibner Ph.D., author of *Vaccination: 100 Years of Orthodox Research shows that Vaccines Represent a Medical Assault on the Immune System* reports that many cases of sudden infant death have post-mortem findings that are similar to Selye's research subjects who died from stress and share similar symptoms of stress prior to death. Some infants could be dying from the stress of vaccinations. Scheibner warns that sudden infant death can occur one month or longer after vaccination.[108]

- Deaths due to immune system disruption. In the immune system section of this chapter, we discussed the possible negative effects that vaccines can have on the immune system. A few studies have linked SIDS to abnormal immune function.[109,110] One study revealed that the diphtheria-tetanus-pertussis vaccine may prevent some unexplained infant deaths due to asymptomatic whooping cough, but it may also initiate an autoimmune reaction which has been implicated in many cases of SIDS.[111] The IOM reviewed this issue of abnormal immune function leading to SIDS and concluded that "there is insufficient information concerning the role of...abnormal inflammatory response leading to sudden unexpected infant death."[112]

- Lack of studies. To my knowledge, there are no studies that explore the possible correlation between administering all the vaccines currently recommended in our pediatric schedule in the same child and the risk of sudden infant death. Ideally, this type of research would use unvaccinated infants as a control group and include follow-ups with children for at least a few months after vaccine administration.

## *Should I worry about mercury in vaccines?*

It has been stated that there is no legitimate safety reason for children, pregnant women, or others to avoid thimerosal-containing vaccines.[113] However, thimerosal is approximately 50% mercury,[114] and mercury is one of the top ten most toxic substances.[115] Since the mid-1990s, efforts have been made to greatly reduce the amount of mercury found in children's vaccines.[116,117] This removal has alleviated concerns regarding the toxicity of children's vaccines. However, thimerosal is still found in some vaccines administered to children and pregnant women in North America and is used to prevent the contamination of vaccines with bacteria and fungi.[118]

In addition to mercury, other vaccine components are also known to be toxic to humans. For example, it has been known for years that aluminum can be toxic to the human nervous system and yet most children's vaccines in North America contain aluminum. Aluminum is added to increase the immune response so that a lesser amount of the active ingredient and fewer doses are used.[119] However, there are conflicting opinions regarding how effective aluminum is at stimulating the immune system in a beneficial manner. Below is a discussion of the concerns regarding the use of mercury and aluminum in children's vaccines.

- Lack of safety guidelines. No guidelines have been developed regarding how much aluminum or mercury is safe to inject into infants and children at repeated intervals throughout their childhood. Research that examines the long-term health effects of repeatedly injecting the combination of potential toxins found in vaccines into infants and children is desperately needed. Ideally, safety guidelines would consider the cumulative dose of potential toxins administered together in a series of vaccines, both the short and long-term health effects of the injection of potential toxins, and the increased susceptibility of infants to the harmful effects of toxins. Safety margins need to be established for infants and children based on relevant research, with as little theoretical extrapolations as possible. Research that investigates the short-term health effects of injecting a single vaccine in adults is insufficient proof that the same combination of potential toxins is safe to repeatedly inject into an infant. Research would even be less relevant if the subjects in the study are ingesting the substance in question instead of having it injected, are exposed to a similar substance instead of the substance commonly used in vaccines, or are injected only once with the substance in question instead of at repeated intervals.

- Children are at a higher risk of toxic effects. Infants and unborn children are more susceptible to toxic effects of mercury on the nervous system.[120,121] Mercury can interfere with the normal neurological development in the offspring of exposed mothers.[122] Fetal exposure to aluminum can result in a higher distribution of aluminum to the brain.[123] Excess aluminum can adversely affect the nervous system, especially if the fetus is exposed during development. Aluminum can be passed on to unborn children and infants through the placenta and through breast milk.[124] Women who avoid exposure to aluminum and mercury during pregnancy and actively remove these substances from their bodies prior to pregnancy, with a medical professional, will decrease their risk of passing these heavy metals on to their children through pregnancy and breastfeeding.

- Health conditions may be due to mercury and/or aluminum accumulation. There is abundant research that denies the connection between mercury and neurological disorders.[125] Other research, however, supports the connection between mercury and neurological disorders.[126,127,128,129] One study concluded that thimerosal-containing vaccines may significantly increase a child's risk of the following:

    - autism,
    - attention deficit disorder (ADD),
    - speech disorders,
    - abnormalities in thinking,
    - personality disorders,
    - tics,
    - speech and language disorders, and
    - neurodevelopment delays.[130]

In high doses, ethyl mercury (the type of mercury used in some vaccines) can cause tremors, spasms, tingling, numbness, irritability, restlessness, difficulty concentrating, decreased memory, depression, loss of coordination, and speech disturbances.[131] Many of these symptoms resemble those found in autistic children, so it has been hypothesized that some cases of autism are actually a form of mercury toxicity.[132] The doses in vaccines may be small, but some people may be more susceptible to the toxic effects of mercury than others.

Here is a list of conditions that aluminum has been implicated in developing:

- Alzheimer's disease,[133]
- Parkinson's disease,[134, 135]
- Lou Gehrig's disease,[136]
- amyotrophic lateral sclerosis (ALS),[137]
- delayed physical maturation,[138]
- encephalopathy (tremors, convulsions, psychosis, changes in speech, and behaviour),[139]
- anemia,[140]
- brittle or soft bones (osteomalacia),[141]
- rickets,[142]
- glucose intolerance,[143]
- cardiac arrest,[144] and
- macrophagic myofasciitis (MMF).[145]

It is noteworthy that some of these conditions have also been reported as vaccine complications. It is also important to be aware of other sources of mercury and aluminum, so that it can be avoided whenever possible in order to reduce your child's cumulative dose of each of these elements. For a list of sources of mercury and aluminum that can be found in your home, see the accompanying workbook *Childhood Vaccinations: Making Informed Decisions*.

Mercury-containing products should be disposed of carefully through approved disposal sites. Exposure to aluminum is inevitable as it is a naturally occurring metal. It is found in air (especially in industrialized areas), food (dairy and grains),[146] water (especially treated water),[147] and soil. However, exposure through different routes will result in different absorption rates. For example, less than 1% of aluminum that is eaten is absorbed by the body,[148] whereas 99% of aluminum that is injected into a muscle moves directly into the bloodstream within an hour.[149]

Whenever possible, avoid unnecessary exposure to aluminum and mercury. This is especially important if you are pregnant or planning a pregnancy and during the first few years of life. As mentioned earlier in this chapter, children are approximately ten times more susceptible to the toxic effects of chemicals because they are less capable of eliminating toxins due to their immature organ systems and also because they eat more, breathe more, and have double the skin surface area than adults do (relative to their body mass), which means that, pound for pound, children are exposed to more toxins than adults in a similar environment.

A complete list of vaccine ingredients is not available and products labelled "mercury not used as a preservative" may still contain mercury in trace amounts as it may be used during the manufacturing process, and not strictly as a preservative.

# CONCLUSION

It is ultimately up to each parent to make decisions about what is best for his or her child. Ideally, parents should be able to make informed decisions based on current and up to date information with the support of their health care provider. Unfortunately, reliable and relevant information about childhood vaccination issues is not always available and support can be difficult to find. This book and the accompanying workbook are intended to facilitate the process of making informed decisions about childhood vaccinations by clarifying current vaccination issues and options, as well as providing information about vaccine-preventable infections, and offering practical guidelines for parents.

Raising a healthy child involves many factors. I encourage parents to make conscious choices about their child's physical health, but also to consider what they can do to promote mental, emotional, and spiritual health as each of these components play a role in the overall health and development of your children.

# ACKNOWLEDGEMENTS

Thank you Kiefer and Sonya Baird RN, who introduced me to childhood vaccination issues. Thank you to my naturopathic clients who have provided me with the focus for this book. Thank you to everyone who has offered insight, editing, support, and feedback, including the following individuals: Tobi Lin B.Sc., ND; Kelly Dobbin, RM, M.A.; Christine Matheson, ND; Tony Bailetti, Ph.D.; Neil Christopher, B.Ed., M.Ed., Ph.D. (cand.); Anna Ziegler, Donna Christopher and Ibi Kaslik, B.A., M.A. A special thank-you to Anne Marie Bourgeois, M.A.; Danny Christopher, B.F.A.; and Keith Christopher Ph.D. Thank you to all of those who helped me complete my research and those who encouraged me along the way. Thank you, again, Danny, for all of your support and for engaging me in so many hours of discussions about childhood vaccines. And thank you, Kalah, for your patience and for inspiring us to make informed decisions about childhood vaccinations.

Finally, I gratefully acknowledge the contributions to our current understanding of childhood vaccination issues provided by the following doctors, authors, and researchers: Sherri Tenpenny, DO; Archie Kalokerinos, MD, Ph.D.; Catherine Diodati, M.A.; Randall Neustaedter, OMD, LAc, CCH; Stephanie Cave, MS, MD, FAAFP; Veira Scheibner, Ph.D.; Alan Clemetson, MD; Mark Geier, MD, Ph.D.; David Geier, MD; Andrew Wakefield, MD; David Lescheid, ND, Ph.D.; Zoltan Rona, MD; Ronald Gold, MD, MPH; Bruce Milliman, ND; Emily Kane, ND; Eileen Stretch, ND; Neil Miller, ND; Glanna Wilde, ND; and the many others.

# RESOURCES

**Vaccine consultations, education, lectures, and support:**

Katia Bailetti B.Sc., EMA, ND
Email: info@drbailetti.com
Website: www.drbailetti.com

Dr. Katia Bailetti provides vaccination consultations and lectures, natural vaccine support and post-vaccination treatment, as well as ongoing pediatric naturopathic services.

Dr. Sherri Tenpenny DO
Website: www.DrTenpenny.com

Dr. Sherri Tenpenny provides vaccination consultations, lectures and support, as well as family medical services with special interest in ASD/autism, children's health, women's health, and a wide variety of chronic pain problems.

**Recommended books:**

*Childhood Vaccinations: Answers to Your Questions* by Katia Bailetti ND

*Childhood Vaccinations: Making Informed Decisions* by Katia Bailetti ND

*Your Child's Best Shot: A Parent's Guide to Vaccination* by Ronald Gold MD

*The Vaccine Guide: Risks and Benefits for Children and Adults* by Randall Neustaedter OMD, Lac, CCH

*What Your Doctor May Not Tell You about Children's Vaccinations* by Dr. Stephanie Cave MD, FAAFP, and Deborah Mitchell

*Vaccines: The Risks, The Benefits, The Choices, a Resource Guide for Parents* by Dr. Sherri Tenpenny DO

*Vaccinations: A Thoughtful Parent's Guide: How to Make Safe, Sensible Decisions About the Risks, Benefits, and Alternatives* by Aviva Jill Romm

*The Vaccine Book: Making the Right Decision for Your Child* by Robert Sears

**National vaccine recommendations:**

Public Health Agency of Canada: www.phac-aspc.gc.ca/im/is-cv/index.html

Centers for Disease Control and Prevention: www.cdc.gov/vaccines/recs/schedules

Australian Department of Health and Aging: www.health.gov.au/internet/immunise/publishing.nsf/content/nips2

European Surveillance Network for Vaccine-Preventable Diseases: www.euvac.net/graphics/euvac/vaccination/iceland.html

Japan's Infectious Disease Surveillance Center: http://idsc.nih.go.jp/vaccine/dschedule/ImmEN-05rev.pdf

**Exemptions:**

**Exemptions by Province**:

Ontario: www.forms.ssb.gov.on.ca/mbs/ssb/forms/ssbforms.nsf/AttachDocsPublish/014-7470-64E~1/$File/7470-64E.doc

Manitoba: written statement from parent suffices

New Brunswick: www.gnb.ca/0000/pol/e/706AB.pdf

Note: In all other provinces, childhood vaccinations are not required for school entry.

**Exemptions by State:**
www.nvic.org/Vaccine-Laws/state-vaccine-requirements.aspx

**Report a vaccination complication:**

Report of Adverse Events Following Immunization: www.phac-aspc.gc.ca/im/pdf/hc4229e.pdf

Vaccine Adverse Event Reporting System: https://vaers.hhs.gov/esub/index

**Travel vaccine information:**

Travel Health Clinics: www.phac-aspc.gc.ca/tmp-pmv/travel/clinic_e.html

Travel Health Information: www.phac-aspc.gc.ca/tmp-pmv/index.html

Travel Health Information: www.cdc.gov/travel

International Travel and Health Interactive Map: http://apps.who.int/tools/geoserver/www/ith/index.html

**Government vaccine information and Canadian Pediatric Society:**

Public Health Agency of Canada: www.phac-aspc.gc.ca/im/index.html

Canadian Pediatric Society: www.caringforkids.cps.ca/immunization/index.htm

Centers for Disease Prevention and Control: www.cdc.gov/od/science/iso

Vaccine Information Statements: www.cdc.gov/vaccines/pubs/vis/default.htm

**Risk awareness and pro-choice organizations:**

Vaccine Risk Awareness Network (VRAN): www.vran.org

National Vaccine Information Center: www.nvic.org

Think Twice: http://thinktwice.com

Parents Requesting Open Vaccine Information (PROVE): www.vaccineinfo.net

**Major manufacturers of pediatric vaccines:**

GlaxoSmithKline Inc www.gsk.ca

Merck Frosst Canada Ltd: www.merck.ca

Sanofi Pasteur Canada: www.sanofipasteur.ca

Wyeth Canada: www.wyeth.ca

GlaxoSmithKline Biologicals: www.gsk-bio.com/english/index.html

Merck & Co., Inc.: www.merck.com

Sanofi Pasteur: www.sanofipasteur.com

Wyeth Pharmaceuticals, Inc.: www.wyeth.com

**Find a naturopathic doctor:**

Canadian Association of Naturopathic Doctors: www.cand.org

American Association of Naturopathic Physicians: www.naturopathic.org

**Legal representation for vaccine injured:**

Think Twice: www.thinktwice.com/lawyers.htm

# ABOUT THE AUTHOR

Katia Bailetti is a mother and licensed naturopathic doctor who offers natural health care for children in Toronto. Before studying naturopathic medicine at the Canadian College of Naturopathic Medicine, Katia completed a degree in Biology at the University of Ottawa and obtained a Paramedic Diploma from Humber College. Her interest in childhood vaccinations began over a decade ago after hearing about a child who suffered a severe reaction to a vaccine. In 2004, Katia began to research vaccinations and quickly realized how overwhelming the topic was, even for a health care professional. This realization prompted Katia to write this book and the accompanying workbook so that other parents could understand vaccination issues and options and make decisions based on accurate, current and relevant information.

In addition to a pediatric naturopathic practice, Dr. Bailetti offers vaccine consultations across Canada, natural vaccine support and post vaccine treatment and vaccine workshops.

She is also developing resources for the Doctor Mom program. This program was created to help parents safely and confidently use natural medicine at home with their children for minor health concerns and to promote child health education.

Katia recently served on the executive committee of the Association of Perinatal Naturopathic Doctors and remains an active member of the Canadian Association of Naturopathic Doctors. Since 1999, Katia has received four awards in recognition of her various volunteer and community-building efforts.

For more information about Katia Bailetti, to schedule a clinic appointment for your child, a vaccination consultation (in person or by phone), workshop or a speaking engagement, please visit www.drbailetti.com. To find out more about purchasing Dr. Bailetti's books and parenting resources, please visit www.doctormom.me.

# *Chapter 1 Endnotes*

1. Public Health Agency of Canada. *Canada Immunization Guide* (7th Edition). Ottawa, ON: Public Works and Government Services Canada; 2006.

2. Public Health Agency of Canada. Frequently Asked Questions – H1N1 Flu Virus. Public Health Agency of Canada website. Available online: www.phac-aspc.gc.ca/alert-alerte/h1n1/faq_rg_h1n1-eng.php. Accessed October 15, 2009.

3. Public Health Agency of Canada. Publicly Funded Immunization Programs in Canada – Routine Schedule for Infants and Children (including special programs and catch-up programs). Public Health Agency of Canada website. Available online: www.phac-aspc.gc.cza/im/ptimprog-progimpt/table-1_e.html. Accessed July 23, 2007.

4. Department of Health and Human Services, Centers for Disease Prevention and Control. (2007). Recommended Immunization Schedule for Persons Aged 0–6 Years, Recommended Immunization Schedules for Persons Aged 7–18 Years. American Academy of Pediatrics website. Available online: www.cispimmunize.org/IZSchedule_Childhood.pdf. Accessed October 9 2009.

5. Public Health Agency of Canada. Immunization Schedules: Recommendations from the National Advisory Committee on Immunization (NACI). Public Health Agency of Canada website. Available online: www.phac-aspc.gc.ca/im/ptimprog-progimpt/table-1-eng.php. Accessed July 17, 2009.

6. Public Health Agency of Canada. National Advisory Committee on Immunization Statement on conjugate meningococcal vaccine for serogroups A, C, Y and W-135. 2007;33(ACS-3):1-24. Available online: www.phac-aspc.gc.ca/publicat/ccdr-rmtc/07pdf/acs33-03.pdf.

7. Centres for Infectious Disease Prevention and Control – Notifiable Diseases Online, notifiable disease incidence by age group [database online]. Public Health Agency of Canada; 2005. Updated April, 2005. Available online: http://dsol-smed.phac-aspc.gc.ca/dsol-smed/ndis/index_e.html.

8. In conversation with Mr. Scott, C., Surveillance Officer (Nosocomial and Occupational Infections Section), Infectious Disease Prevention and Control, Public Health Agency of Canada (March 2007).

9. Centres for Infectious Disease Prevention and Control– Notifiable Diseases Online, notifiable disease incidence by age group [database online]. Public Health Agency of Canada; 2005. Updated April, 2005. Available online: http://dsol-smed.phac-aspc.gc.ca/dsol-smed/ndis/index_e.html.

10. Public Health Agency of Canada. National Advisory Committee on Immunization Statement on Human Papillomavirus Vaccine. *Canada Communicable Diseases Report*. 2007;33(ACS-2):1–25. Available online: www.phac-aspc.gc.ca/publicat/ccdr-rmtc/07pdf/acs33-02.pdf.
11. Ibid.

12. Public Health Agency of Canada. Canadian National Report on Immunization. November 2006; 32S3. Available online: www.phac-aspc.gc.ca/publicat/ccdr-rmtc/06vol32/32s3/index-eng.php.
13. Ibid.

14. Public Health Agency of Canada. Update on the Invasive Meningococcal Disease and Meningococcal Vaccine Conjugate Recommendations. *Canada Communicable Disease Report.* 2009;35(ACS-3):1-40. Available online: www.phac-aspc.gc.ca/publicat/ccdr-rmtc/09vol35/acs-dcc-3/index-eng.php. Accessed October 24, 2009.
15. Ibid.

16. Public Health Agency of Canada. Guidance Document on the Use of Pandemic Influenza A (H1N1) 2009 Inactivated Monovalent Vaccine. October 21, 2009. Available online: www.phac-aspc.gc.ca/alert-alerte/h1n1/vacc/pdf/monovacc-guide-eng.pdf. Accessed January 15, 2010.
17. Ibid.

18. Public Health Agency of Canada. Surveillance: Deaths associated with H1N1 flu virus in Canada. Public Health Agency of Canada website. Available online: www.phac-aspc.gc.ca/alert-alerte/h1n1/surveillance-archive/20100107-eng.php. Accessed January 15, 2010. Accessed January 7, 2010.

19. Statistics Canada. Mortality, Summary List of Causes, 2003. Catalogue no. 84F0209XIE. Available online: http://dsp psd.pwgsc.gc.ca/Collection/Statcan/84F0209X/84F0209XIE2003000.pdf. Accessed January 7, 2010.

20. Statistics Canada. Mortality, Summary List of Causes, 2004. Catalogue no. 84F0209XI. Available online: http://dsp-psd.pwgsc.gc.ca/collection_2007/statcan/84F0209X/84F0209XIE2004000.pdf. Accessed January 7, 2010.

21. Statistics Canada. Mortality, Summary List of Causes, 2005. Available online: www.statcan.gc.ca/pub/84f0209x/2005000/tablcsectlist-listetableauxsect-eng.htm. Accessed January 7, 2010.

22. Public Health Agency of Canada. Frequently Asked Questions – H1N1 Flu Virus. Public Health Agency of Canada website. Available online: www.phac-aspc.gc.ca/alert-alerte/h1n1/faq_rg_h1n1-eng.php. Accessed October 24, 2009.

23. Public Health Agency of Canada. Overall Influenza Summary Week 26 (September 6 to 12 2009). Public Health Agency of Canada website. Available online: www.phac-aspc.gc.ca/fluwatch/09-10/w36_09/pdf/fw2009-36-eng.pdf. Accessed October 15, 2005.

24. Public Health Agency of Canada. Overall Influenza Summary Week 36 (September 6 to 12 2009). Public Health Agency of Canada website. Available online: www.phac-aspc.gc.ca/fluwatch/09-10/w36_09/pdf/fw2009-36-eng.pdf. Accessed October 15, 2005.

25. World Health Organization. Influenza: Seasonal: April 2009. World Health Organization website. Available online: www.who.int/mediacentre/factsheets/fs211/en/. Accessed January 15, 2010.

26. Public Health Agency of Canada. *Canada Immunization Guide* (7th Edition). Ottawa, ON: Public Works and Government Services Canada; 2006.

27. US National Library of Medicine and National Institutes of Health. Measles. Medical Encyclopedia, Medline Plus website. Available online: www.nlm.nih.gov/medlineplus/ency/article/001569.htm. Accessed August 18, 2006.

28. US National Library of Medicine and National Institutes of Health. Mumps. Medical Encyclopedia, Medline Plus website. Available online: www.nlm.nih.gov/medlineplus/ency/article/001557.htm. Accessed August 18, 2006.

29. US National Library of Medicine and National Institutes of Health. Rubella. (Medical Encyclopedia, Medline Plus website. Available online: www.nlm.nih.gov/medlineplus/ency/article/001574.htm. Accessed May 1, 2007.

30. US National Library of Medicine and National Institutes of Health. Varicella. Medical Encyclopedia, Medline Plus website. Available online: www.nlm.nih.gov/medlineplus/ency/article/001592.htm. Accessed July 26, 2007.

31. US National Library of Medicine and National Institutes of Health. Influenza. Medical Encyclopedia, Medline Plus website. Available online: www.nlm.nih.gov/medlineplus/ency/article/000080.htm. Accessed January 18, 2006.

32. US National Library of Medicine and National Institutes of Health. Viral Gastroenteritis. Medical Encyclopedia, Medline Plus website. Available online: www.nlm.nih.gov/medlineplus/ency/article/000252.htm. Accessed February 14, 2007.

33. US National Library of Medicine and National Institutes of Health. Hepatitis A. Medical Encyclopedia, Medline Plus website. Available online: www.nlm.nih.gov/medlineplus/ency/article/000278.htm. Accessed July 28, 2006.

34. US National Library of Medicine and National Institutes of Health. Human Papillomavirus Vaccine. Medical Encyclopedia, Medline Plus website. Available online: www.nlm.nih.gov/medlineplus/druginfo/medmaster/a607016.html. Accessed April 1, 2007.

35. US National Library of Medicine and National Institutes of Health. Diphtheria. Medical Encyclopedia, Medline Plus website. Available online: www.nlm.nih.gov/medlineplus/ency/article/001608.htm. Accessed September 25, 2007.

36. US National Library of Medicine and National Institutes of Health. Tetanus. Medical Encyclopedia, Medline Plus website. Available online: www.nlm.nih.gov/medlineplus/ency/article/000615.htm. Accessed November 27, 2006.

37. US National Library of Medicine and National Institutes of Health. Pertussis. Medical Encyclopedia, Medline Plus website. Available online: www.nlm.nih.gov/medlineplus/ency/article/001561.htm. Accessed March 2, 2006.

38. US National Library of Medicine and National Institutes of Health. Poliomyelitis. Medical Encyclopedia, Medline Plus website. Available online: www.nlm.nih.gov/medlineplus/ency/article/001402.htm. Accessed March 6, 2006.

39. Public Health Agency of Canada. *Canada Immunization Guide* (7th Edition). Ottawa, ON: Public Works and Government Services Canada; 2006.

40. Public Health Agency of Canada. Vaccine-Preventable Diseases: *Haemophilus Influenzae* type B. Public Health Agency of Canada website. Available online: www.phac-aspc.gc.ca/im/vpd-mev/hib-eng.php. Accessed Oct. 20 2009.

41. US National Library of Medicine and National Institutes of Health. Meningitis-H.Influenzae. Medical Encyclopedia, Medline Plus website. Available online: www.nlm.nih.gov/medlineplus/ency/article/000612.htm. Accessed September 6, 2006.

42. Public Health Agency of Canada. *Canada Immunization Guide* (7th Edition). Ottawa, ON: Public Works and Government Services Canada; 2006.

43. Ibid.

44. US National Library of Medicine and National Institutes of Health. Measles. Medical Encyclopedia, Medline Plus website. Available online: www.nlm.nih.gov/medlineplus/ency/article/001569.htm. Accessed August 18, 2006.

45. Public Health Agency of Canada. *Canada Immunization Guide* (7th Edition) Ottawa, ON: Public Works and Government Services Canada; 2006.
46. Ibid.
47. Ibid.

48. US National Library of Medicine and National Institutes of Health. Rubella. Medical Encyclopedia, Medline Plus website. Available online: www.nlm.nih.gov/medlineplus/ency/article/001574.htm. Accessed May 1, 2007.

49. Public Health Agency of Canada. *Canada Immunization Guide* (7th Edition). Ottawa, ON: Public Works and Government Services Canada; 2006.

50. US National Library of Medicine and National Institutes of Health. Meningococcal meningitis. Medical Encyclopedia, Medline Plus website. Available online: www.nlm.nih.gov/medlineplus/ency/article/000608.htm. Accessed August 15, 2006.
51. Ibid.

52. US National Library of Medicine and National Institutes of Health. Pneumococcal meningitis. Medical Encyclopedia, Medline Plus website. Available online: www.nlm.nih.gov/medlineplus/ency/article/000607.htm. Accessed August 15, 2006.

53. Public Health Agency of Canada. *Canada Immunization Guide* (7th Edition). Ottawa, ON: Public Works and Government Services Canada; 2006.

54. US National Library of Medicine and National Institutes of Health. Pneumococcal meningitis. Medical Encyclopedia, Medline Plus website. Available online: www.nlm.nih.gov/medlineplus/ency/article/000607.htm. Accessed August 15, 2006.

55. Public Health Agency of Canada. *Canada Immunization Guide* (7th Edition). Ottawa, ON: Public Works and Government Services Canada; 2006.

56. US National Library of Medicine and National Institutes of Health. Influenza. Medical Encyclopedia, Medline Plus website. Available online: www.nlm.nih.gov/medlineplus/ency/article/000080.htm. Accessed January 18, 2006.

57. US National Library of Medicine and National Institutes of Health. Hepatitis *B*. Medical Encyclopedia, Medline Plus website. Available online: www.nlm.nih.gov/medlineplus/ency/article/000279.htm. Accessed January 23, 2006.

58. US National Library of Medicine and National Institutes of Health. Genital Warts. Medical Encyclopedia, Medline Plus website. Available online: www.nlm.nih.gov/medlineplus/ency/article/000886.htm. Accessed February 8, 2007.

59. US National Library of Medicine and National Institutes of Health. Viral Gastroenteritis. Medical Encyclopedia, Medline Plus website. Available online: www.nlm.nih.gov/medlineplus/ency/article/000252.htm. Accessed February 14, 2007.

60. US National Library of Medicine and National Institutes of Health. Hepatitis A. Medical Encyclopedia, Medline Plus website. Available online: www.nlm.nih.gov/medlineplus/ency/article/000278.htm. Accessed July 28, 2006.

61. Public Health Agency of Canada. *Canada Immunization Guide* (7th Edition). Ottawa, ON: Public Works and Government Services Canada; 2006.
62. Ibid.

63. Statistics Canada. Mortality, Summary List of Causes, 2004 Census. Statistics Canada website. Available online: www.statcan.ca/english/freepub/84F0209XIE/84F0209XIE2004000.pdf. Accessed August 10, 2007.

64. Statistics Canada. Mortality, Summary List of Causes, 2005 Census. Statistics Canada website. Available online: www.statcan.gc.ca/pub/84f0209x/84f0209x2005000-eng.pdf. Accessed September 30, 2009.

65. Statistics Canada. Mortality, Summary List of Causes, 2004 Census. Statistics Canada website. Available online: www.statcan.ca/english/freepub/84F0209XIE/84F0209XIE2004000.pdf. Accessed August 10, 2007.

66. Statistics Canada. Mortality, Summary List of Causes, 2005 Census. Statistics Canada website. Available online: www.statcan.gc.ca/pub/84f0209x/84f0209x2005000-eng.pdf Accessed September 30, 2009.

67. Cancer Society of Canada.The human papillomavirus (HPV) and cervical cancer. Canadian Cancer Society website. Available online: www.cancer.ca/ccs/internet/standard/0,3182,3649_1242735771__langId-en,00.html. Accessed March 7, 2007.

68. Statistics Canada. Age and Sex Highlight Tables, 2006 Census. Statistics Canada website. Available online: www12.statcan.ca/english/census06/data/highlights/agesex/websites/website.cfm?Lang=E&Geo=PR&Code=01&Table=3&Data=Count&Sex=1&StartRec=1&Sort=2&Display=website. Accessed August 10, 2007.

69. Statistics Canada. Mortality, Summary List of Causes, 2004 Census. Statistics Canada website. Available online: www.statcan.ca/english/freepub/84F0209XIE/84F0209XIE2004000.pdf. Accessed August 10, 2007.
70. Ibid.

71. Public Health Agency of Canada. *Canada Immunization Guide* (7th Edition). Ottawa, ON: Public Works and Government Services Canada; 2006.
72. Ibid.

73. Public Health Agency of Canada. Vaccine Preventable Diseases, Immunization and Vaccines. Public Health Agency of Canada website. Available online: www.phac-aspc.gc.ca/im/vpd-mev/index.html. Accessed May 23, 2007.

74. US National Library of Medicine and National Institutes of Health. Meningococcal meningitis. Medical Encyclopedia, Medline Plus website. Available online: www.nlm.nih.gov/medlineplus/ency/article/000608.htm. Accessed August 8, 2006.

75. US National Library of Medicine and National Institutes of Health. Pneumococcal meningitis. Medical Encyclopedia, Medline Plus website. Available online: www.nlm.nih.gov/medlineplus/ency/article/000607.htm. Accessed August 15, 2006.

76. Public Health Agency of Canada. *Canada Immunization Guide* (7th Edition). Ottawa, ON: Public Works and Government Services Canada; 2006.
77. Ibid.
78. Ibid.

79. US National Library of Medicine and National Institutes of Health. Human Papillomavirus Vaccine. Medical Encyclopedia, Medline Plus website. Available online: www.nlm.nih.gov/medlineplus/druginfo/medmaster/a607016.html. Accessed April 1, 2007.
80. Ibid.

81. Public Health Agency of Canada. National Advisory Committee on Immunization Statement on Human Papillomavirus Vaccine. Canada Communicable Diseases Report. 2007;33(ACS-2):1-25. Available online: www.phac-aspc.gc.ca/publicat/ccdr-rmtc/07pdf/acs33-02.pdf

82. US National Library of Medicine and National Institutes of Health. Human Papillomavirus Vaccine. Medical Encyclopedia, Medline Plus website. Available online: www.nlm.nih.gov/medlineplus/druginfo/medmaster/a607016.html. Accessed April 1, 2007.

83. Public Health Agency of Canada. *Canada Immunization Guide* (7th Edition). Ottawa, ON: Public Works and Government Services Canada; 2006.
84. Ibid.

85. US National Library of Medicine and National Institutes of Health. Hepatitis B. Medical Encyclopedia, Medline Plus website. Available online: www.nlm.nih.gov/medlineplus/ency/article/000279.htm. Accessed January 23, 2006.
86. Ibid.

87. US National Library of Medicine and National Institutes of Health. Diphtheria. Medical Encyclopedia, Medline Plus website. Available online: www.nlm.nih.gov/medlineplus/ency/article/001608.htm. Accessed September 25, 2007.

88. US National Library of Medicine and National Institutes of Health. Tetanus. Medical Encyclopedia, Medline Plus website. Available online: www.nlm.nih.gov/medlineplus/ency/article/000615.htm. Accessed November 27, 2006.

89. US National Library of Medicine and National Institutes of Health. Pertussis. Medical Encyclopedia, Medline Plus website. Available online: www.nlm.nih.gov/medlineplus/ency/article/001561.htm. Accessed March 2, 2006.

90. US National Library of Medicine and National Institutes of Health. Meningitis-H.Influenzae. Medical Encyclopedia, Medline Plus website. Available online: www.nlm.nih.gov/medlineplus/ency/article/000612.htm. Accessed September 6, 2006.

91. US National Library of Medicine and National Institutes of Health. Meningococcal meningitis. Medical Encyclopedia, Medline Plus website. Available online: www.nlm.nih.gov/medlineplus/ency/article/000608.htm. Accessed August 15, 2006.

92. US National Library of Medicine and National Institutes of Health. Pneumococcal meningitis. Medical Encyclopedia, Medline Plus website. Available online: www.nlm.nih.gov/medlineplus/ency/article/000607.htm. Accessed August 15, 2006.

93. US National Library of Medicine and National Institutes of Health. Diphtheria. Medical Encyclopedia, Medline Plus website. Available online: www.nlm.nih.gov/medlineplus/ency/article/001608.htm. Accessed September 25, 2007.

94. US National Library of Medicine and National Institutes of Health. Tetanus. Medical Encyclopedia, Medline Plus website. Available online: www.nlm.nih.gov/medlineplus/ency/article/000615.htm. Accessed November 27, 2006.

95. Public Health Agency of Canada. *Canada Immunization Guide* (7th Edition). Ottawa, ON: Public Works and Government Services Canada; 2006.

96. Public Health Agency of Canada. Poliomyelitis. Public Health Agency of Canada (Notifiable Diseases) website. Available online: http://dsol-smed.phac-aspc.gc.ca/dsol-smed/ndis/disease2/poli_e .html. Accessed January 20, 2006.

97. US National Library of Medicine and National Institutes of Health. Meningitis-H.Influenzae. Medical Encyclopedia, Medline Plus website. Available online: www.nlm.nih.gov/medlineplus/ ency/article/000612.htm. Accessed September 6, 2006.

98. Public Health Agency of Canada. Vaccine-Preventable Diseases: *Haemophilus Influenzae* type B. Public Health Agency of Canada website. Available online: www.phac-aspc.gc.ca/im/vpd-mev/hib-eng.php. Accessed Oct. 20 2009.

99. Public Health Agency of Canada. Definitions of high risk for three new publicly funded vaccines by Province/Territory. Public Health Agency of Canada website. Available online: www.phac-aspc.gc.ca/ im/ptimprog-progimpt/table-5_e.html. Accessed April 3, 2007.

100. Public Health Agency of Canada. Update on the Invasive Meningococcal Disease and Meningococcal Vaccine Conjugate Recommendations. *Canada Communicable Disease Report*. 2009;35(ACS-3):1-40. Available online: www.phac-aspc.gc.ca/ publicat/ccdr-rmtc/09vol35/acs-dcc-3/index-eng.php. Accessed October 24, 2009.

101. Health Canada. Pneumococcal Vaccine – It's Your Health. Health Canada website. Available online: www.hc-sc.gc.ca/hl-vs/iyh-vsv/ med/pneum-eng.php. Accessed October 24, 2009.

102. Public Health Agency of Canada. Definitions of high risk for three new publicly funded vaccines by Province/Territory. Public Health Agency of Canada website. Available online: www.phac-aspc.gc.ca/im/ptimprog-progimpt/table-5_e.html. Accessed April 3, 2007.

103. US National Library of Medicine and National Institutes of Health. Influenza. Medical Encyclopedia, Medline Plus website. Available online: www.nlm.nih.gov/medlineplus/ency/article/000080.htm. Accessed January 18, 2006.

104. Centers for Disease Control and Prevention. Interim Guidance for Clinicians on Identifying and Caring for Patients with Swine-origin Influenza A (H1N1) Virus Infection. Centers for Disease Control and Prevention website. Available online: www.cdc.gov/h1n1flu/identifyingpatients.htm. Accessed October 24, 2009.

105. Canadian Broadcasting Corporation. Seasonal Flu Shot May Increase H1N1 Risk. Canadian Broadcasting Corporation website. Available online: www.cbc.ca/health/story/2009/09/23/flu-shots-h1n1-seasonal.html. Accessed October 24, 2009.

106. Public Health Agency of Canada. *Canada Immunization Guide* (7th Edition). Ottawa, ON: Public Works and Government Services Canada; 2006.

107. US National Library of Medicine and National Institutes of Health. Genital Warts. Medical Encyclopedia, Medline Plus website. Available online: www.nlm.nih.gov/medlineplus/ency/article/000886.htm. Accessed February 8, 2007.

108. US National Library of Medicine and National Institutes of Health. Viral Gastroenteritis. Medical Encyclopedia, Medline Plus website. Available online: www.nlm.nih.gov/medlineplus/ency/article/000252.htm. Accessed February 14, 2007.

109. US National Library of Medicine and National Institutes of Health. Hepatitis A. Medical Encyclopedia, Medline Plus website. Available online: www.nlm.nih.gov/medlineplus/ency/article/000278. Accessed July 28, 2006.

## *Chapter 2*

1. In Conversation with Ms. Sonja Baird, mother of Kiefer (January 20th, 2007).

2. Fombonne E., Zakarian R., Bennett, McLean-Heywood D. Pervasive Developmental Disorders in Montreal, Quebec, Canada: Prevalence and Links with Immunizations. *PEDIATRICS*. 2006;118(1): 139–150.

3. Public Health Agency of Canada.National Consensus Conference on Pertussis. *Canada Communicable Disease Report.* 2003;29S3(3). Available online: www.phac-aspc.gc.ca/publicat/ccdr-rmtc/07vol33/dr3313b-eng.php

4. Public Health Agency of Canada.Frequently Asked Questions H1N1 Flu Virus. Public Health Agency of Canada website. Available online: www.phac-aspc.gc.ca/alert-alerte/h1n1/faq_rg_h1n1-eng.php#vac

5. Public Health Agency of Canada. Vaccine Safety: Surveillance of Adverse Events Following Immunization. Canadian National Report on Immunization, 2006 [taken from *Canada Communicable Disease Report*]. November 2006;32S3. Available online: www.phac-aspc.gc.ca/publicat/ccdr-rmtc/06vol32/32s3/5vacc-eng.php. Accessed January 7, 2010.
6. Ibid.
7. Ibid.
8. Ibid.

9. Ontario Ministry of Health and Long Term Care. Publicly Funded Immunization Schedules for Ontario–February 2005. Ontario Ministry of Health and Long Term Care website. Available online: www.health.gov.on.ca/english/providers/program/immun/pdf/schedule.pdf. Accessed February 2005.

10. Public Health Agency of Canada. *Canada Immunization Guide* (7th Edition). Ottawa, ON: Public Works and Government Services Canada; 2006.

11. Public Health Agency of Canada. *Canada Immunization Guide* (7th Edition). Ottawa, ON: Public Works and Government Services Canada;2006.

12. Agency for Toxic Substances and Disease Registry. Formaldehyde. Agency for Toxic Substances and Disease Registry 1999 website. Available online: www.atsdr.cdc.gov/tfacts111.pdf. Accessed February 2005.

13. Rosenthal S, Chen R. The Reporting Sensitivities of Two Passive Surveillance Systems for Vaccine Adverse Events: Public Health Briefs. *American Journal of Public Health.* 1995;85(12):1706–1709.

14. Public Health Agency of Canada. *Canada Immunization Guide* (7th Edition). Ottawa, ON: Public Works and Government Services Canada;2006.

15. Public Health Agency of Canada. Vaccine Safety (Canadian Adverse Events Following Immunization Surveillance System). Public Health Agency of Canada website. Available online: www.phac-aspc.gc.ca/im/vs-sv/caefiss_e.html. Accessed November 11, 2006.

16. Public Health Agency of Canada. *Canada Immunization Guide* (7th Edition). Ottawa, ON: Public Works and Government Services Canada; 2006.
17. Ibid.
18. Ibid.

19. Bhandari M., Busse J.W., Jackowski D., et.al. Association between industry funding and statistically significant pro-industry findings in medical and surgical randomized trials. *Canadian Medical Association Journal.* 2004;170(4):477-80.

20. Lexchin J., Bero L.A., Djulbegovic B., Clark O. Pharmaceutical industry sponsorship and research outcome and quality: systematic review. *British Medical Journal.* 2003;326(7400):1167–1170.

21. Public Health Agency of Canada. *Canada Immunization Guide* (7th Edition). Ottawa, ON: Public Works and Government Services Canada; 2006.
22. Ibid.
23. Ibid.

24. Clemetson A.B. Vaccinations, Inoculations and Ascorbic Acid. *Journal of Orthomolecular Medicine.* 1999;4(3):137–142.

25. Tenpenny S. *Vaccines, What CDC Documents and Science Reveal* [DVD]. Cleveland, OH: New Medical Awareness Seminars; 2003.

26. Diodati C. *Immunization – History, Ethics, Law and Health.* Windsor, ON: Integral Aspects, Inc.;1999.

27. Public Health Agency of Canada. *Canada Immunization Guide* (7th Edition) Ottawa, ON: Public Works and Government Services Canada; 2006.

28. Shulman LM. Oral polio vaccine: will it help eradicate polio or cause the next epidemic? *The Israel Medical Association Journal.* 2006;8(5)312–315.

29. Public Health Agency of Canada. *Canada Immunization Guide* (7th Edition). Ottawa, ON: Public Works and Government Services Canada; 2006.
30. Ibid.
31. Ibid.

32. US Health Resources and Services Administration. National Vaccine Injury Compensation Program. US Department of Health and Human Services website. Available online: www.hrsa.gov/vaccinecompensation/table.htm. Accessed August 24, 2007.

33. Public Health Agency of Canada. *Canada Immunization Guide* (7th Edition). Ottawa, ON: Public Works and Government Services Canada; 2006.

34. Brown D. Vaccine Failure Is Setback in AIDS Fight–Test Subjects May Have Been Put at Extra Risk Of Contracting HIV. *Washington Post.* March 21, 2008. www.washingtonpost.com/wp-dyn/content/article/2008/03/20/AR2008032003398.html?hpid=topnews&sid=ST2008032101286. Accessed March 21, 2008.

35. Mulholland EK. Measles in the United States, 2006. *New England Journal of Medicine.* 2006;355(5):440–443.

36. Lee B.R., Feaver S.L., Miller C.A., Hedberg C.W., Ehresmann KR. An Elementary School Outbreak of Varicella Attributed to Vaccine Failure: Policy Implications. *Journal of Infectious Diseases.* 2004;190(3):477–483.
37. Ibid.
38. Ibid.

39. Public Health Agency of Canada *Canada Immunization Guide* (7th Edition). Ottawa, ON: Public Works and Government Services Canada; 2006.
40. Ibid.

41. Jefferson T. Influenza vaccination: policy versus evidence. *British Medical Journal.* 2006;333(7574):912–915.

42. Trotter C.L.. Antibody to Haemophilus influenzae type b after routine and catch-up vaccination. *Lancet.* 2003;361(9368):1523–1524.

43. Raguckas SE. Pertussis resurgence: diagnosis, treatment, prevention and beyond. *Pharmacotherapy.*2007;27(1):41–52.

44. Sokhin A.A. Duration of the preservation of postvaccinal immunity against measles and the results of a repeat immunization of children with various initial antibody levels [abstract]. *Zhurnal Mikrobiologii, Epidemiologii, I Immunobiologii.*1983;PMID(Sep-9-6 637278):79–85.

45. Borrow R. Long-term protection in children with meningococcal C conjugate vaccination: lessons learned. *Expert Review Of Vaccines.* 2006;(6):851–857.

46. Linder N., Vishne T.H., Levin E., et al. Hepatitis B Vaccination: Long-term Follow-up of the Immune Response of Preterm Infants and Comparison of Two Vaccination Protocols. *Infection.*2002;30(3):136-139.

47. Gillum J.E. Current Immunization Practices. *Postgraduate Medicine.* 1989;85(2)183–186, 188–190, 195–198.
48. Ibid.
49. Ibid.

50. Mulholland K. Measles in the United States. *The New England Journal of Medicine.* 2006;355(5):440–443.

51. Caro J.J. Economic burden of pertussis and the impact on immunization. *The Pediatric Infectious Disease Journal.* 2005;24(Suppl 5):S48–54.

52. Stratton K., Almario D., McCormick, M. *Immunization Safety Review: SV40 Contamination of Polio Vaccine and Cancer.* Washington, D.C.: The National Academies Press; 2002.

53. Horowitz L.G. *Emerging Viruses: AIDS & Ebola: Nature, Accident or Intentional.* Rockport, Massachusetts: Tetrahedron Publishing Group; 1997.

54. US National Library of Medicine, National Institutes of Health. Creutzfeldt-Jakob disease. Medical Encyclopedia, Medline Plus website. Available online: www.nlm.nih.gov/medlineplus/ency/article/000788.htm. Accessed September 7, 2006.

55. Gherardi R.K., Coquet M., Cherin P., et al. Macrophagic myofasciitis lesions assess long-term persistence of vaccine-derived aluminium hydroxide in muscle. *Brain.* 2001;124(Pt. 9):1821–1831.
56. Ibid.
57. Ibid.
58. Ibid.

59. CBC News. Seasonal Flu Shot May Increase H1N1 Risk. CBC News website. Available online: www.cbc.ca/health/story/2009/09/23/flu-shots-h1n1-seasonal.html. Accessed September 23, 2009.

60. Public Health Agency of Canada. Canadian National Report on Immunization,1996. [taken from *Canada Communicable Disease Report*]. May 1997;23S4. Available online: www.phac-aspc.gc.ca/publicat/ccdr-rmtc/97vol23/23s4/index.html. Accessed January 8, 2010.

61. Public Health Agency of Canada. *Canada Immunization Guide* (7th Edition). Ottawa, ON: Public Works and Government Services Canada; 2006.

62. Ibid.

63. Ibid.

64. Buxbaum S. Epidemiological analysis of immunity against vaccine-preventable diseases: rubella, measles, mumps and chickenpox [abstract]. *Deutsche Medizinische Wochenschrift.* 2001;126(46)1289–1293.

65. Moalem S., Prince J. *Survival of the Sickest.* New York, NY: HarperCollins; 2007.

66. Relman D.A. The Human Body as a Microbial Observatory. *Nature Genetics.* 2002;30(2):131–133.

67. Moalem S., Prince J. *Survival of the Sickest.* New York, NY: HarperCollins; 2007.

68. Canadian Institute for Health Research and Health Canada. Biological Terrorism – Canadian Research Agenda. Viral Agents Panel Presentation; January 19, 2002; Toronto, ON.

69. Public Health Agency of Canada. National Immunization Strategy. *Final Report 2003.* Ottawa, ON: Public Works and Government Services Canada; 2003.

70. Merck & Co. Inc. 2005 Annual Report. *Financial Section.* Whitehouse Station, NJ; 2005. Available online: www.merck.com/finance/annualreport/ar2005/financial_section.html. Accessed January 8, 2010.

71. Daubs K. Former CMAJ editors launch advertising-free medical journal *Ottawa Citizen.* April 18, 2007. www.canada.com/ottawacitizen/news/city/story.html?id=62b28112-3a4b-4c45-bb83-2b40a89700de. Accessed April 18, 2007.
72. Ibid.

73. Maskalyk J. Why Open Medicine? *Open Medicine.* 2007;1(1). Available online: www.openmedicine.ca/article/view/74/3

74. Wilson K, Barakat M, Mills E, et al. Addressing the emergence of pediatric vaccination concerns: Recommendations from a Canadian policy analysis. *Canadian Journal of Public Health.* 2006;97(2)139–141.

75. US Health Resources and Services Administration. National Injury Compensation Program. Vaccination Injury Compensation website. Available online: www.hrsa.gov/vaccinecompensation/. Accessed August 25, 2007.
76. Ibid.

## *Chapter 3*

1. Canadian Society of Allergy and Clinical Immunology. About the Society. Canadian Society of Allergy and Clinical Immunology website. Available online: www.csaci.medical.org. Accessed August 8, 2007.
2. Ibid.

3. Statistics Canada. Persons with arthritis or rheumatism, by age group and sex. (1994–2005). Statistics Canada website. Available online: www40.statcan.ca/l01/cst01/health51a.htm. Accessed August 13, 2007.

4. Multiple Sclerosis Society of Canada. Medical Update Memo. Multiple Sclerosis Society of Canada website. Available online:www.mssociety.ca/en/research/pdf/medmmo-sexratio-20061031.pdf#xml=www.mssociety.ca/SCRIPTS/texis.exe/webinator/search/pdfhi.txt?query=increasing+incidence&pr=default&prox=page&rorder=500&rprox=500&rdfreq=500&rwfreq=500&rlead=500&sufs=0&order=r&cq=&id=4548621678. Accessed October 31, 2007.

5. Gillespie KM. Type 1 diabetes: pathogenesis and prevention. Canadian Medical Association Journal. 2006;175(2):165–170.

6. Multiple Sclerosis Society of Canada. Multiple sclerosis is a complex disease. Multiple Sclerosis Society of Canada website. Available online: www.mssociety.ca/en/information/default.htm. Accessed August 26, 2007.

7. Tishler M., Shoenfeld Y. Vaccination may be associated with autoimmune diseases. *The Israel Medical Association Journal.* 2004;6(7):430–432.

8. Matricardi P.M., Bonini S. Mimicking microbial 'education' of the immune system: a strategy to revert the epidemic trend of atopy and allergic asthma? *Respiratory Research.* 2000;1(3):129–132.

9. Anway D Matthew, Skinner K Michael. Epigenetic Trans-generational Actions of Endocrine Disruptors. *Endocrinology.* Jun 2006;147:s43–s49.

10. Hurwitz E.L., Morgenstern H.E. Effects of diphtheria-tetanus-pertussis or tetanus vaccination on allergies and allergy-related respiratory symptoms among children and adolescents in the United States. *Journal of Manipulative Physiological Therapeutics.* 2000;23(2):81–90.
11. Ibid.

12. Tishler M., Shoenfeld Y. Vaccination may be associated with autoimmune diseases. The Israel Medical Association Journal. 2004;6(7):430–432.

13. Olesen, A.B. Atopic dermatitis is increased following vaccination for measles, mumps and rubella or measles infection. *Acta Dermato-Venereologica* [abstract]. 2003;83(6):445–450.

14. Tishler M., Shoenfeld Y. Vaccination may be associated with autoimmune diseases. *The Israel Medical Association Journal.*2004;6(7):430–432.

15. Shoenfeld Y., Aron-Maor A. Vaccination and Autoimmunity – 'Vaccinosis': A Dangerous Liaison? *Journal of Autoimmunity.* 2000;14(1):1–10.

16. Tishler M., Shoenfeld Y. Vaccination may be associated with autoimmune diseases. *The Israel Medical Association Journal.* 2004; 6(7):430–432.
17. Ibid.
18. Ibid.
19. Ibid.
20. Ibid.
21. Ibid.

22. Shoenfeld Y., Aron-Maor A. Vaccination and Autoimmunity – 'Vaccinosis': A Dangerous Liaison? *Journal of Autoimmunity.* 2000;14(1):1–10.

23. Lescheid D. Childhood Vaccinations and Immunity: A Naturopathic Perspective. *Vital Link: Canadian Association of Naturopathic Doctors.* 2005;12(2):1–10.

24. Stratton K., Wilson C. *Immunization Safety Review: Multiple Immunizations and Immune Dysfunction.* Washington, DC: National Academy Press; 2006. http:// www.nap.edu/catalog/10306.html. Accessed April 8, 2007.

25. Lescheid D. Childhood Vaccinations and Immunity: A Naturopathic Perspective. *Vital Link: Canadian Association of Naturopathic Doctors.* 2005; 12(2):1–10.
26. Ibid.
27. Ibid.
28. Ibid.
29. Ibid.

30. Ogra P.L., Faden H, Welliver RC. Vaccination Strategies for Mucosal Immune Responses. *Clinical Microbiology Reviews.* 2001;14(2):430-445.

31. Seipp R. Mucosal Immunity and Vaccines. *The Science Creative Quarterly* 2007;Jan–March 2007(2):S45-S53.

32. Lescheid D. Childhood Vaccinations and Immunity: A Naturopathic Perspective. *Vital Link: Canadian Association of Naturopathic Doctors.* 2005;12(2):1–10.

33. Modlin J.F., Halsey N.A., Thoms M.L., Meschievitz C.K., Patriarca P.A. Humoral and mucosal immunity in infants induced by three sequential inactivated poliovirus vaccine-live attenuated oral poliovirus vaccine immunization schedules. *Journal of Infectious Diseases.* 1997;175 (suppl 1):S228–S234.

34. Public Health Agency of Canada. Immunization Schedules: Recommendations from the National Advisory Committee on Immunization (NACI).Public Health Agency of Canada website. Available online: www.phac-aspc.gc.ca/im/ptimprog-progimpt/table-1-eng.php. Accessed July 17, 2009.

35. Public Health Agency of Canada. *Canada Immunization Guide* (7th Edition). Ottawa, ON: Public Works and Government Services Canada;2006.
HPV reference: Public Health Agency of Canada. National Advisory Committee on Immunization Statement on Human Papillomavirus Vaccine. *Canada Communicable Diseases Report.* 2007;33(ACS-2):1-25. Available online: www.phac-aspc.gc.ca/publicat/ccdr-rmtc/07pdf/acs33-02.pdf

36. Public Health Agency of Canada. *Canada Immunization Guide* (7th Edition). Ottawa, ON: Public Works and Government Services Canada; 2006.

37. Public Health Agency of Canada. National Advisory Committee on Immunization Statement on Human Papillomavirus Vaccine. *Canada Communicable Diseases Report 2007*. 2007;33(ACS-2):1–25. Available online: www.phac-aspc.gc.ca/publicat/ccdr-rmtc/07pdf/acs33-02.pdf.

38. Crinnion W. Environmental Medicine, Part 1: The Human Burden of Environmental Toxins and Their Common Health Effects. *Alternative Medicine Review.* 2000;5(1):52–63.

39. Page G.G. Are There Long-term Consequences of Pain in Newborn or Very Young Infants? *Journal of Perinatal Education.* 2004;13(3)10–17.

40. Stratton K., Almario D.A., McCormick M.C. *Immunization Safety Review: SV40 Contamination of Polio Vaccine and Cancer.* Washington, DC: National Academy Press; 2002.
41. Ibid.

42. Public Health Agency of Canada. Polio Vaccine and SV40, Questions and Answers. Public Health Agency of Canada website. Available online: www.phac-aspc.gc.ca/im/polio_e.html. Accessed April 8, 2007.

43. Stratton K, Almario D.A., McCormick M.C. *Immunization Safety Review: SV40 Contamination of Polio Vaccine and Cancer.* Washington, DC: National Academy Press; 2002.
44. Ibid.
45. Ibid.

46. Kyle W.S. Simian retroviruses, poliovaccine and origin of AIDS. *Lancet.* 1992;339(8793):600-601.

47. Horowitz L.G. Polio, hepatitis B and AIDS: an integrative theory on a possible vaccine induced pandemic. *Medical Hypotheses.* 2001;56(5):677–686.

48. Horby P. Variant Creutzfeldt-Jakob disease: an unfolding epidemic of misfolded proteins. *Journal Of Paediatrics And Child Health.* 2002;38(6):539–542.
49. Ibid.

50. Public Health Agency of Canada. CJD–SS Progress Report, CJD in Canada, Annual Update 2006. Public Health Agency of Canada website. Available online: www.phac-aspc.gc.ca/hcai-iamss/cjd-mcj/cjdss-ssmcj/pdf/newsletter06_e.pdf. Accessed April 9, 2007.

51. National Institute of Neurological Disorders and Stroke. Creutzfeldt-Jakob Disease Fact Sheet. National Institute of Neurological Disorders and Stroke website. Available online: www.ninds.nih.gov/disorders/cjd/detail_cjd.htm. Accessed April 9, 2007.

52. Public Health Agency of Canada. CJD–SS Progress Report, CJD in Canada, Annual Update 2006. Public Health Agency of Canada website. Available online: www.phac-aspc.gc.ca/hcai-iamss/cjd-mcj/cjdss-ssmcj/pdf/newsletter06_e.pdf. Accessed April 9, 2007.

53. US National Library of Medicine, National Institutes of Health. Creutzfeldt-Jakob Disease. Medical Encyclopedia, Medline Plus website. Available online: www.nlm.nih.gov/medlineplus/ency/article/000788.htm. Accessed September 7, 2006.

54. Erstad B.L. Implications of prion-induced diseases for animal-derived pharmaceutical products. *American Journal of Health-System Pharmacy*. 2002;59(3):254–263.

55. Public Health Agency of Canada. *Canada Immunization Guide* (7th Edition). Ottawa, ON: Public Works and Government Services Canada; 2006.

56. US Food and Drug Administration. Bovine Spongiform Encephalopathy (BSE). US Food and Drug Administration website. Available online: www.fda.gov/cber/BSE/risk.htm. Accessed April 8, 2007.

57. Norris, S. Potential Causes of Autism Spectrum Disorders. Library of Parliament, Parliamentary Information and Research Service, Science and Technology Division. February 23rd, 2006. Available online: www2.parl.gc.ca/Content/LOP/ResearchPublications/prb0587-e.pdf.

58. Wakefield A.J., Murch S.H., Anthony A., et al. Ileal-lymphoid-nodular hyperplasia, nonspecific colitis, and pervasive developmental disorder in children. *Lancet.* 1998;351(9103):637–641.

59. Immunization Safety Review Committee. *Immunization Safety Review: Vaccines and Autism.* Washington, DC: National Academy Press; 2004.
60. Ibid.

61. Public Health Agency of Canada. Vaccine Safety: Frequently Asked Questions. Public Health Agency of Canada website. Available online: www.phac-aspc.gc.ca/im/vs-sv/vs-faq_e.html#11. Accessed October 18, 2005.

62. Wakefield A.J. Vaccines and Autism: Enterocolitis, autism and measles virus. Molecular Psychiatry. 2002;7:S44–S46. 2010._18 .pdf.

63. Wakefield A., Montgomery S. Autism, Viral Infection and Measles-Mumps-Rubella Vaccination. *Israel Medical Association Journal.* 1999;1:183–187.
64. Ibid.
65. Ibid.
66. Ibid.

67. Finegold S.M., Molitoris D., Song Y., et. al. Gastrointestinal Microflora Studies in Late-Onset Autism. *Clinical Infectious Diseases.* 2002;35 (suppl 1):S6-S16.

68. Geier D.A., Geier M.R.. A two-phased population epidemiological study of the safety of thimerosal-containing vaccines: a follow up analysis. Medical Science Monitor. 2005 Apr;11(4):CR160–70

69. Public Health Agency of Canada. Exposure to Thimerosal in Vaccines used in Canadian Infant Immunization Programs, with Respect to risk of Neurodevelopmental Disorders. *Canada Communicable Disease Report 2002.* 2002;28(09). Available online: www.phac-aspc.gc.ca/publicat/ccdr-rmtc/02vol28/dr2809ea.html.
70. Ibid.

71. Bernard S., Enayati A., Redwood L., Roger H., Binstock T.. Autism: a novel form of mercury poisoning. *Medical Hypotheses.* 2001;56(4):462–471.

72. Geier D.A. A clinical trial of combined anti-androgen and anti-heavy metal therapy in autistic disorders. *Neuro Endocrinology Letters.* 2006;27(6):833–838.

73. Autism Research Institute. Parent Ratings of Behavorial Effects of Biomedical Interventions. Autism Research Institute website. Available online: www.autism.com/treatable/form34qr.htm. Accessed August 27, 2007.

74. Muran P.J. Mercury Elimination with Oral DMPS, DMSA, Vitamin C and Glutathione: An Observational Clinical Review. *Alternative Therapies in Health & Medicine.* 2006;12(3):70–75.

75. Public Health Agency of Canada. Vaccine Safety: Surveillance of Adverse Events Following Immunization 2006. *Canada Communicable Disease Report 2006*. November, 2006;32S3:29–35. Available online: www.phac-aspc.gc.ca/publicat/ccdr-rmtc/06pdf/32s3_e.pdf

76. Immunization Safety Review Committee. Immunization Safety Review: Vaccines and Autism. Washington, DC: National Academy Press; 2004.

77. Blaylock R. Interaction of Cytokines, Excitotoxins, and Reactive Nitrogen and Oxygen Species in Autism Spectrum Disorders. *Journal of the American Neutraceutical Association*. 2003;6(4);21–35.

78. US Department of Health and Human Services. Statistics. National SIDS/Infant Death Resource Center website. Available online: www.sidscenter.org/Statistics.aspx?fromparent=parent&id=6&heading=Statistics. Accessed February 2, 2007.

79. Canadian Foundation for The Study of Infant Deaths. Number of SIDS deaths in Canada 1990–2003. Sudden Infant Death Syndrome (Canada) website. Available online: www.sidscanada.org/sidsnews.htm. Accessed November 15, 2005.

80. US Department of Health and Human Services. Statistics. National SIDS/Infant Death Resource Center website. Available online: www.sidscenter.org/Statistics.aspx?fromparent=parent&id=6&heading=Statistics. Accessed February 2, 2007.
81. Ibid.

82. Canadian Foundation for The Study of Infant Deaths. Number of SIDS deaths in Canada 1990–2003. Sudden Infant Death Syndrome (Canada) website. Available online: www.sidscanada.org/sidsnews.htm. Accessed November 11, 2005.

83. Stratton K., Almario D.A., Wizemann T.M., McCormick M.C. *Immunization Safety Review: Vaccinations and Sudden Unexpected Death in Infancy*. Washington, DC: National Academy Press; 2003.
84. Ibid.
85. Ibid.

86. Public Health Agency of Canada. Vaccine Safety: Frequently Asked Questions. Public Health Agency of Canada website. Available online: www.phac-aspc.gc.ca/im/vs-sv/vs-faq_e.html#11. Accessed October 18, 2005.

87. US Department of Health and Human Services. Statistics. National SIDS/Infant Death Resource Center website. Available online: www.sidscenter.org/Statistics.aspx?fromparent=parent&id=6&heading=Statistics. Accessed February 2, 2007.

88. Canadian Foundation for The Study of Infant Deaths. Number of SIDS deaths in Canada 1990–2003. Sudden Infant Death Syndrome (Canada) website. Available online: www.sidscanada.org/faq.htm www.sidscanada.org/sidsnews.htm. Accessed August 28, 2007.

89. Public Health Agency of Canada. Vaccine Safety: Surveillance of Adverse Events Following Immunization 2006. *Canada Communicable Disease Report 2006*. November 2006;32S3:29–35. Available online: www.phac-aspc.gc.ca/publicat/ccdr-rmtc/06pdf/32s3_e.pdf.
90. Ibid.
91. Ibid.

92. United States Department of Health and Human Services, Vaccine Adverse Event Reporting System (VAERS), CDC WONDER online database. http://wonder.cdc.gov/vaers.html. Updated December 30, 2009. Accessed January 11, 2010.
93. Ibid.

94. Ahmad SR. Adverse Drug Event Monitoring at the Food and Drug Administration, (Your Report Can Make a Difference). *Journal of General Internal Medicine.* 2003;18(1):57–60.

95. United States Department of Health and Human Services, Vaccine Adverse Event Reporting System (VAERS), CDC WONDER online database. http://wonder.cdc.gov/vaers.html. Updated December 30, 2009. Accessed January 11, 2010.

96. US Department of Health and Human Services. Statistics. National SIDS/Infant Death Resource Center website. Available online: www.sidscenter.org/Statistics.aspx?fromparent=parent&id=6&heading=Statistics. Accessed February 2, 2007.

97. Ottaviani G., Archiv V. Sudden infant death syndrome (SIDS) shortly after hexavalent vaccination: another pathology in suspected SIDS? *An International Journal Of Pathology.* 2006;448(1):100–104.

98. Ibid.

99. The National Center on Shaken Baby Syndrome. Answers to Shaken Baby Syndrome Questions. The National Center on Shaken Baby Syndrome website. Available online: http://dontshake.com/Audience.aspx?categoryID=7&PageName=MedicalFactsAnswers.htm. Accessed August 28, 2007.

100. Clemetson A. Caffey Revisited: A Commentary on the Origin of "Shaken Baby Syndrome." *Journal of Physicians and Surgeons.* 2006;11(1):78–80.

101. Ibid.

102. Ibid.

103. Clemetson C.A. Vaccinations, inoculations and ascorbic acid. *Journal of Orthomolecular Medicine.* 1999;14:137–142.

104. Clemetson A. Caffey Revisited: A Commentary on the Origin of "Shaken Baby Syndrome." *Journal of Physicians and Surgeons.* 2006;11(1):20–21.

105. Ibid.

106. King W.J, MacKay M., Angela Sirnick A. Shaken baby syndrome in Canada: clinical characteristics and outcomes of hospital cases. *Canadian Medical Association Journal.* 2003;168(2):155–159.

107. Selye H. *The Stress of Life.* New York, NY: The McGraw-Hill Companies, Inc.; 1978.

108. Scheibner V. Dynamics of critical days as part of the dynamics of non-specific stress syndrome discovered during monitoring with Cotwatch breathing monitor. *Journal of the Australian College of Nutrition and Environmental Medicine.* 2004;23(3):1–5.

109. Raza M.W, Blackwell C.C. Sudden infant death syndrome, virus infections and cytokines [abstract]. *FEMS Immunology Medical Microbiology.* 1999;25(1–2):85–96.

110. Vege A., Rognum T.O. Sudden infant death syndrome, infection and inflammatory responses [abstract]. FEMS Immunology & Medical Microbiology. 2004;42(1):3–10.

111. Essery S.D. The protective effect of immunisation against diphtheria, pertussis and tetanus (DPT) in relation to sudden infant death syndrome. *FEMS Immunology And Medical Microbiology.* 1999;25(1–2):183–92.

112. Stratton K., Almario D.A., Wizemann T.M., McCormick M.C. *Immunization Safety Review: Vaccinations and Sudden Unexpected Death in Infancy.* Washington, DC: National Academy Press; 2003.

113. National Advisory Committee on Immunization. Updated Recommendations on the use of Thimerosal-Containing Vaccines in Canada. *Canada Communicable Disease Report 2005.* 2005;31(ACS–12):1–4. Available online: www.phac-aspc.gc.ca/publicat/ccdr-rmtc/05pdf/acs-dcc3112.pdf.

114. Public Health Agency of Canada. Exposure to Thimerosal in Vaccines used in Canadian Infant Immunization Programs, With Respect to Risk of Neurodevelopmental Disorders. *Canada Communicable Disease Report 2002.* 2002;29–09. Available online: www.phac-aspc.gc.ca/publicat/ccdr-rmtc/02vol28/dr2809ea.html.

115. US Department of Health and Human Services. Toxicological Profile for Mercury. Agency for Toxic Substances and Disease Registry; March 1999. Available online: www.atsdr.cdc.gov/toxprofiles/tp46.pdf. Accessed January 11, 2010.

116. Public Health Agency of Canada. Exposure to Thimerosal in Vaccines used in Canadian Infant Immunization Programs, With Respect to Risk of Neurodevelopmental Disorders. *Canada Communicable Disease Report 2002.* 2002;28(09). Available online: www.phac-aspc.gc.ca/publicat/ccdr-rmtc/02vol28/dr2809ea.html.

117. Public Health Agency of Canada. Statement on Thimerosal. *Canada Communicable Disease Report 2003.* 2003;29 (ACS 1):1–10.

118. Public Health Agency of Canada. *Canada Immunization Guide* (7th Edition Ottawa, ON: Public Works and Government Services Canada; 2006.

119. Ibid.

120. US Department of Health and Human Services. Toxicological Profile for Mercury. Agency for Toxic Substances and Disease Registry; March 1999. Available online: www.atsdr.cdc.gov/toxprofiles/tp46.pdf. Accessed January 11, 2010.

121. Public Health Agency of Canada. Exposure to Thimerosal in Vaccines used in Canadian Infant Immunization Programs, With Respect to Risk of Neurodevelopmental Disorders. *Canada Communicable Disease Report 2002.* 2002;29–09.

122. US Department of Health and Human Services. Toxicological Profile for Mercury. Agency for Toxic Substances and Disease Registry; March 1999. Available online: www.atsdr.cdc.gov/toxprofiles/tp46.pdf. Accessed January 11, 2010.

123. US Department of Health and Human Services. Public Health Service. Draft Toxic Substances and Disease Registry. Toxicological Profile for Aluminum; September 2008. Available online: www.atsdr.cdc.gov/toxprofiles/tp22.pdf. Accessed January 11, 2010.

124. Ibid.

125. Immunization Safety Review Committee. *Immunization Safety Review: Vaccines and Autism.* Washington, DC: National Academy Press; 2004.

126. Crinnion W.J. Environmental medicine, part three: long-term effects of chronic low-dose mercury exposure. *Alternative Medicine Review.* 2000;5(3):209–223.

127. Bradstreet J., Geier D.A., Kartzinel J.J., Adams J.B., Geier M.R. A Case-Control Study of Mercury Burden in Children with Autistic Spectrum Disorders. *Journal of American Physicians and Surgeons.* 2003;8(3):76–79.

128. Geier D.A., Geier M.R.. Early Downward Trends in Neurodevelopmental Disorders Following Removal of Thimerosal-Containing Vaccines. *Journal of American Physicians and Surgeons.* 2006;11(1): 8–13.

129. Bradstreet J., Geier D.A., Kartzinel J.J., Adams J.B., Geier M.R. A Case-Control Study of Mercury Burden in Children with Autistic Spectrum Disorders. *Journal of American Physicians and Surgeons.* 2003;8(3):76–79.

130. Ibid.

131. Public Health Agency of Canada. Exposure to Thimerosal in Vaccines used in Canadian Infant Immunization Programs, with Respect to risk of Neurodevelopmental Disorders. *Canada Communicable Disease Report 2002.* 2002;28–09. Available online: www.phac-aspc.gc.ca/publicat/ccdr-rmtc/02vol28/dr2809ea.html.

132. Ibid.

133. Health Canada. Aluminum and human health (Environmental and Workplace Health). Health Canada website. Available online: www.hc-sc.gc.ca/ewh-semt/water-eau/drink-potab/aluminum-aluminium_e.html. Accessed March 20, 2006.

134. Ibid.

135. US Department of Health and Human Services. Public Health Service. Draft Toxic Substances and Disease Registry. Toxicological Profile for Aluminum; September 2008. Available online: www.atsdr.cdc.gov/toxprofiles/tp22.pdf. Accessed January 11, 2010.

136. Health Canada. Aluminum and human health (Environmental and Workplace Health). Health Canada website. Available online: www.hc-sc.gc.ca/ewh-semt/water-eau/drink-potab/aluminum-aluminium_e.html. Accessed March 20, 2006.

137. US Department of Health and Human Services. Public Health Service. Draft Toxic Substances and Disease Registry. Toxicological Profile for Aluminum; September 2008. Available online: www.atsdr.cdc.gov/toxprofiles/tp22.pdf. Accessed January 11, 2010.

138. Ibid.

139. Health Canada. Aluminum and human health (Environmental and Workplace Health). Health Canada website. Available online: www.hc-sc.gc.ca/ewh-semt/water-eau/drink-potab/aluminum-aluminium_e.html. Accessed March 20, 2006.

140. Ibid.

141. Health Canada. Aluminum and human health (Environmental and Workplace Health). Health Canada website. Available online: www.hc-sc.gc.ca/ewh-semt/water-eau/drink-potab/aluminum-aluminium_e.html. Accessed March 20, 2006.

142. Ibid.

143. Ibid.

144. Ibid.

145. Gherardi R., Coquet M., Cherin P., et al. Macrophagic myofasciitis lesions assess long-term persistence of vaccine-derived aluminum hydroxide in muscle. *Brain.* 2001;124(9):1821–1831.

146. Health Canada. *Aluminum and human health (Environmental and Workplace Health).* Health Canada website. Available online: www.hc-sc.gc.ca/ewh-semt/water-eau/drink-potab/aluminum-aluminium_e.html. Accessed March 20, 2006.

147. Nayak P. Perinatal Toxicity Of Aluminum. *The Internet Journal of Toxicology* [serial online]. 2006;3(1). Available online: www.ispub.com/ostia/index.php?xmlFilePath=journals/ijto/vol3n1/aluminum.xml. Accessed March 20, 2006.

148. Health Canada. Aluminum and human health (Environmental and Workplace Health). Health Canada website. Available online: www.hc-sc.gc.ca/ewh-semt/water-eau/drink-potab/aluminum-aluminium_e.html. Accessed March 20, 2006.

149. Priest N.D. The biological behaviour and bioavailability of aluminum in man, with special reference to studies employing aluminium-26 as a tracer: review and study update. *Journal of Environmental Monitoring.* 2004;6(5):375–403.